Wings to Freedom

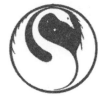

By
Yogiraj Satgurunath Siddhanath

wings to freedom

By Yogiraj Satgurunath Siddhanath

Published by Hamsa Yoga Sangha, Revised Edition 2011

Cover Photograph by Atul Sharma

Printed in INDIA

Photos

Our thanks to all those who have kindly provided their photographs for this work. Unless otherwise indicated, all photos are from *Yogiraj Siddhanath's* personal collection. **At the request of his devotees, a variety of photos of *Gurunath* were included to show the *Satguru* in his various *avastas* (states) and attires.** Som and Rita Bakshi have provided Himalayan Photos.

DEDICATED TO

Babaji

THE HEART OF DIVINITY

THROBBING IN HUMANITY

Contents

Note to the Reader

It is both an honor and a privilege to present this inspirational and informative spiritual masterpiece, from a contemporary representative of the timeless Nath Masters of Yoga. Through his remarkable experiences, and deep insights, Yogiraj Gurunath Siddhanath has made accessible the perennial philosophy of peace and liberation from the deathless Himalayan Masters, in simple, direct and concrete terms. He is always guided by the light of that Being, who defies all limitations, variously known as "The Ancient of Days," or "The Great Sacrifice," and whom Yogiraj calls Shiva-Goraksha-Babaji.

This inter-weaving of formative experiences, with the penetrating wisdom of an enlightened Master, has been a labor of love spanning a period of almost five years in his busy schedule of service to humanity. Everyone who has spent time with *Yogiraj* can testify to his *siddhis*, or spiritual powers, but due to his innate humility, and wish for his readers to focus on the message of peace, rather than sensationalizing his miraculous healing and spiritual powers, such testimonies have been omitted. *Yogiraj* lets his spiritual powers manifest as necessary for helping or teaching others. The only example included is an incident which testifies to the efficacy of his Solar *Yoga*, which was reported in the newspaper.

We would like to express our thanks to the many disciples in the USA and India who have helped edit, design, and refine the book over the years, in the sincere spirit of service to the *Guru* and to humanity, including but not limited to: Rita Bakshi, Runbir Singh, Sylvia Stanley, Kamaljeet Kaur, Ellen Sarbonne, Doug Varn, Bryan Gates, Daniel Kogan, Jay Ponti and Matthew Samowitz, with whose gracious service this book has become so beautiful. It should also be noted that *Yogiraj* labored over every aspect of this book from beginning to end in full effort to share his experiences with the world.

It is our sincere wish that the wisdom of *Yogiraj Gurunath Siddhanath* offered in this work will assist all sincere seekers of Truth along their journey to Self-realization.

— *Gurunath Sanatana Yoga (Hamsa Yoga Sangh)*

CHAPTER 1

COSMIC REBIRTH
My First Meeting with the Immortal Babaji

In the year 1967, I was on my quest to meet the Great Presence called Shiva-Goraksha-Babaji. People call him by many names but He is ever the same, the visible invisible Savior of our Humanity. I made my way up from the holy confluence of Rudraprayag to the sacred city of Badrinath partly by foot and partly by hitch hiking.

Along the way, as I walked amidst the sylvan surroundings of the pines, a breeze wafted by and I recalled past life memories of my yogic endeavors in the Himalayas. The aroma of the pine cones and berries crushed under my feet as I walked along unbeaten trails. My sojourn was so intoxicating that I couldn't contain my nostalgia and so was transferred to a more expansive sense of unity with nature.

The evening sunsets, of many hues of gold, crimson and green came, making the trees throw their lengthening shadows on the meadows. These were followed by the morning sun, dazzling the Alakananda river, to greet me as I woke up. The whole ambience was a meditation. I myself was a meditation and as I sat in deep love of Babaji, a fresh mountain breeze blew through me, bringing its inspiring message that, "the Soul is immortal and the body a boat to ferry us across to this realization." My mind lost its reason in a stream of intuition as I scribbled out my joy:

Déjà vu

In wooded valleys berries crushed
The flavor of the mystic musk
Within me did old memories rise
Devotions to the sunset skies

Forest aroma deep in damp
Wild smell of the wooded pines
Oh! The déjà vu of jungle times
Of long past meditations lives

Where in sylvan bowers I sat
Not in this world nor in that
Just in the joy of Selfing mirth
The odor of the fragrant earth!

My mind a laughing gurgling stream
Running the bedrocks mossy green
Becomes a calm meandering dream
Flowing into Myself serene

With body dead consciousness live
Expanding in eternal skies
Beyond Maya's conditioned dream
The self merging in Self supreme.

"Oh Lord," I prayed, "thought have such deep heart roots in Bharat*," give me the spiritual wings to fly to Thee. Make me the eternal *Hamsa* (swan), for when I look at the stark rugged peaks rising one higher than the other, range after range, it reminds me of the

---

* The land whose people are wedded to the Light of the Soul.

tapa and mighty Yoga of the Nath Yogis. I cannot make it lest you give me a helping hand. Give me the strength, Oh Amarnath Goraksha!"

I carried on walking and bathing in the rivers till I reached Badrinath, the sacred playground of Shiva and Parvati. It is said that Narayana, in the form of a child, was found by Parvati, who looked after him and Shiva blessed Narayana to stay at this place and use it for his Lila and meditation. The Lord Narayana and Nara are established in meditation for the welfare of the World. They are Krsna and Arjuna respectively. But esoterically, the divine Cosmic Being Krsna Narayana is meditating for the welfare and evolution of Nara, representing the whole of humanity.

Badrinath Temple, dedicated to Lord Narayana, is at a height of 10,500 feet, tucked away in winter amidst the Himalayan snows. The temple stands at the foot of the majestic Neelakanta Mountain, dedicated to Lord Shiva, which soars to about 25,000 feet or more. Its snow capped peak is usually covered by clouds. Flanked by the two mountains, Sonar Suli and Narayana, on a clear day the Neelakanta Peak looks like a snow diamond.

I tarried at Badrinath a few days to acclimatize. During those days I visited the Temple of Badrinath to meditate. On my *pradakshina* (clockwise circling of the temple), I saw a most awe inspiring painting of the monumental *Siddha* with his matted dreadlocks covered with the snow; each *rudraksha* bead of his *mala* had a hint of snow. Yes, this was he, whose photo I had in my underground meditation room in Sinhagad, Pune. This was none other than the majestic Raja Sundernath.

I stood in awe, lost in admiration of this Divine Yogi of the Gorakshanath lineage. He was recently, in 1924, the *Mahant* (head) of Goraknath temple at Gorakpur, which is of the *Dharam-Nath* sub-sect of Goraknath Yogis. Sundernath is the same yogi who entered the body of a South Indian cow-herd and became the *Siddha* Tirumoolar who wrote the famous treatise on Yoga, *Thiru-mandiram*. This

3

Himalayan Yogi Raja Sundernath is still alive in his *Sanjeevan* body at Alkapuri on the Indo-China border.

The Nath, established in *Svaroop Samadhi*, is truly the likes of whom saved India's spiritual heritage from the fate that befell ancient Egypt, Babylon, China, Tibet, and the Mayan civilization of South America. India is alive even today as it was ten thousand years ago. It is the spiritual dynamo of the world today, destined to lead the material world to its haven of spiritual Truth in the coming new age. Many of these ancient spiritual cultures have been long since dead. Not only this, but from time immemorial such *Siddha Nath* yogis have been the guardian wall of our humanity and guardians of the Himalayan peaks, according to popular belief. The classical pose of this Yogi depicting India's past and present glory threw me into glorious trance. Nowhere else in the world has there been a lifestyle where a yogi sacrifices his all in his quest for God, not caring where his next meal is coming from, putting his life on the line. His passion for God consumes his entire life and transforms him into the Divine Superman like Goraknath and other sages who have gone before him in "robes of light." He pursues the Divine with single-minded purpose. Travelling on foot from Kedarnath to Badrinath, often going hungry, the pilgrim and ascetic gives his all to seek his beloved Lord. The yogi possesses nothing yet owns the world.

After I came to myself from this reverie, I proceeded onwards to Charan Paduka, another holy stop where Rama, the seventh *avatar* of Vishnu had rested during his sojourn in the Himalayas.

The cave I call "*Jhilmilee Gufa*" is located at the foot of the Neelakanteswar ("blue-throated" Shiva) Mountain. The route was a beaten trail, which became steeper. As I walked into the silence, my awareness became deeper. It was as if I was entering a heavenly sphere, which indeed it was. A different dimension this was, as I trod lightly and breathed a different air so crisp and other worldly.

As my trek to the sacred cave continued, I felt a strong urge to look back. There I saw a young girl. I still remember that scene, so vividly impressed in my mind. She may have been anything from twelve to fourteen. She wore this *ghagara-chunari* (a colorful large skirt and veil), and had a fair and rosy complexion like the Himachal apple. She was standing with a sickle in one hand, with the other on her hips. As I looked at her, I became a child and asked her, "Don't you feel afraid here all alone in the vast Himalayan mountains?" She smiled at me and I thought I'd become a two-year-old child. I thought, "Am I asking the proper question to the proper person? I mean, who am I asking this question to?" She stood with such confidence as if the whole world belonged to her, her hair flowing freely over her back and shoulders. I knew in my sub-conscious mind that she, who had a most unearthly aura about her, was an aspect of the Divine Mother, but I was not bringing myself to believe this.

I told myself, "You know that this is true. It is the Divine Mother in her *Kanya* form," which means a small girl of twelve. I asked, "Do you know the way to Babaji's cave?" She just ignored my question and said, "Everything will be well and all. Be happy. See, I am happy." So, I turned around thinking that if she's not bothering to answer my question, why should I bother to ask about the road.

Nothing really matters. If nothing really matters why not go where the breeze takes you. So I went in the direction of the breeze. Crazy....I was out of my mind. I didn't know what dimension I was in. But I knew I was not in a physical or emotional state of mind. I was in a totally different awareness altogether. I don't remember which of the trips this was (there was another little girl with me) whether it was the first time I went or the second time. She gave me some latex, which is found between the bark of the tree and its inner skin. As my breath was heavy, I chewed it and my tiredness went away. I was fresh again.

After a few steps I looked around and there was nobody there, no one around. The divine girl just vanished. I cursed myself for not having recognized her and grabbing her feet and asking for her blessings. I didn't even do the *pranam* because she'd thrown the veil of *maya* on me so that I couldn't recognize who she was. It was only after she disappeared that she allowed it to dawn on me that she was an aspect of the Goddess, who was guiding my footsteps to the cave of Babaji. I felt very, very exhilarated and disappointed, all at the same time. I carried on my ascent to the cave of Babaji, I knew not where.

As I traveled on I became more convinced that Babaji is Lord Shiva himself. When I reached the top I was tired and exhausted. I saw the whole Himalayan range from the lower mountains near the cave, and it was like the laughter of Shiva, the teeth of Shiva, all along the range from one end to the other. I came to a gentle slope and felt as if I could glide off and fly off into eternal space, above the snow-capped mountains beyond the clouds.

I was very exhausted and lay on my back for a breather, as the setting sun went behind the clouds. It became chilly and dark. After a while, from behind the clouds, another light appeared and I did not know what it was. "Ah! The sun has come back," I thought to myself. My thoughts were answered by a voice, "Indeed, if you think it is the sun, it is." I saw a great shimmering light filling the whole area. I saw the essence of the light, the spiritual aura; the spiritual feel of the whole scene was of another world. It may be Babaji. It may not be Babaji. Who it is I do not know, I cannot say.

I felt it was not proper for me to be on my back. So with great effort, I turned on my stomach and did the *shastanga pranam* (salutation by joining both hands and prostrating on the ground). Lost in wonder and in awe, I asked him, "Who are you?" I asked the Nameless Being, this Great Presence. And from this word an ode sprung forth like a fountain.

Who art thou? I know thee not.
And yet I am of thee
I cannot comprehend thee, Lord
Thou Emperor of Divinity

I sit and melt in silence
Of thy love, O Infinite
Make me thy Truth
Make me thy Love
Eternal Lord of Light

He said, "Whoever thou thinkest me to be, that I am for thee". Even though my ego, my emotions are limited to Shiva, Ganapati, Christ, and Buddha, he is beyond the Christ and the Buddha because he is "Non-being Essentially". Our understanding is limited and so is our thinking, because he is so vast that he is nothing. But he is the source of everything. Even if you were to take everything out from him, he would still be complete.

Om purnamada purnamidam
Purnat purna mudachyatae
Purnasya purna madaya
Purna meva vashisyathae

This is what he was! I could not capacitate his voltage. So I saw him from my past life association with him, and my lips took the proper shape and my voice said "Shiva-Goraksha-Babaji". No sooner had I said this, then his voice rang out in the firmament of my heart and in the surrounding mountains, *"Tathastu, Tathastu!"*

The connection with Shiva Gorakshanath was the memory in my super-conscious mind. He wanted to pull my desire out of my own memory bank so that the word would come from me and not from him, as to who he was, who this Eternal Now was. He would not comment. As Shiva-Goraksha-Babaji has gone beyond the "rings pass not," with no possibility of his return to our world cycle, his being with us on the planet is a stupendous mystery.

If I said Allah, it would be Allah. If I said Ganapati, it would be Ganapati. He wanted to pull out from my memory bank my *karmic* life with him from my past lives. Therefore he waited for an answer from me. I said, "Who art Thou? I know Thee not and yet I am of Thee." He said, "Who you thinkest me to be, that I am to thee! I am That I am!" He was non-being, egoless, the formless, eternal unborn Self who had no identity, not as any human understanding is concerned.

Then I found a cold wave running from the top of my head to my toes. It was a cold and warm sort of current, you know. It was a cold wave coming up from the bottom of my feet to the top of my head, and a warm wave washing my body from the top of my head to my toes. Then the process reversed itself. It was as though I was being revamped and cleansed.

I thought after ten, twelve hours of meditation a person's *nadis* would be cleansed and he would be pure to receive him. In my own voice he replied, "This is true, but you have to go to a higher level of *samadhi*, which you have not achieved as yet. You will be given this Divine state of realization due to past good *samskaras* and *karmas*. This preparation is therefore necessary for brain and body."

I moved out of my body after the experience of hot and cold, as though my whole body was doing the *Shiva-Shakti* breathing. I do not know how long it lasted. I was totally oblivious of the time. There was no time or space continuum. I was just absorbed by this other worldly bliss and light. I do not know where my eyes were or what is meant by eyes. I moved out of my physical body and expanded into the emotional body. Then after some time the emotional body expanded into the mental body. Then the mental body expanded into the Soul Consciousness. My crystal soul dissolved and expanded into awareness, which was boundless. It seemed like I was undergoing a gentle series of transformative implosions to expand the essence of my Being!

All at once, the trees, the birds, the clouds, the sky, the planets, the stars and the galaxies were me and were breathing my breath and *prana*. The sun's rays were me. There was this vast unity in diversity. It was only then that I was able to capacitate the message given by the

Nameless Being whom the world knows as Babaji whom I, due to my past associations with him as Shiva-Goraksha-Babaji, was able to experience.

It is difficult to describe his form. His hair touched his heels and was ablaze with a radiant fire. His countenance had a heavenly luster and his body appeared wet as though he had had a bath in the Alakhananda river, and yet was dry. He wore a black buck skin with a *kamandalu* in his hand. I perceived that his feet were not touching the ground, but were a few inches above it. As my consciousness familiarized with his Cosmic Consciousness, I felt the oneness of all creation in him. The deathless fragrance of his body told me the tale of his immortality.

Even in *samadhi*, I was thunderstruck, dumbfounded by his spiritual majesty. His Consciousness expanded beyond the seven infinities, and my consciousness expanded to merge in an infinitesimal part of his, I was lost and died unto eternity.

Later, as this soul returned after the experience of both his form and formless Self, I felt, "Oh Lord! The universe, a bubble in my consciousness, my consciousness a nothing in Thy Nothingness! Such is Thine ineffable majesty, no mortals, no angels, can describe. Oh Thou highest of the high, of the Angelic hierarchy of the heavenly host. Thou art all the heavenly host and yet beyond them. Only the Lord God may comprehend Thee, oh Lord, thou about Whom naught may be said!"

This message was not in words. It was in photons of light. His message came to me in shafts of light, in photons, sparks, whatever you call it. I do not know, I do not know the words, but it came to me so fast that volumes were encapsulated in those shafts, in those photons of light, the message to humanity. The message of my serving humanity, becoming the servant of humanity, which is the most honored thing that could happen to me. My *karma* encoded in my DNA was being released to match this experience and support it, but the Divine experience far surpassed my good *karma*. It was pure blessings of the Great One.

It is important to know that I was receiving this information in my super-consciousness, without the participation of my mind. I can say my analytical mind lay subservient to my super-conscious *avasta*. A great lesson was learned—that the analytical mind was an inferior instrument for education and should only be used in daily life for absorbing practical knowledge. The true means for gathering Divine Knowledge is that of a vigilant Consciousness, which gathers true wisdom and gnosis.

Babaji Goraksha, the greatest *Raja Yogi* who ever walked the earth, in his compassion for humanity created the Science of *Hatha Yoga* as a stepping-stone, making thereby an easier approach to *Raja Yoga*. Let not people of feeble minds interpret and limit Shiva-Gorakshanath as a *Hatha Yogi* alone. My journeys entailed many a solitary expedition to places and caves graced by the most magnificent presences. Traveling and meditating alone had its rewards of a ceaseless river of peace flowing through me, and clarifying my mind to visualize and experience higher realms of consciousness, which I would not have been able to avail of myself with more people around.

Even at that time, I was not ready, not capacitated, but due to his grace, I was able to get this experience. This mighty Being called the "Nameless One," the "Lightning Standing Still," was the head, the heart, the seed, and the Soul of undying Knowledge, spread from eternity to eternity, beyond infinity. He could not be understood, only experienced.

It seemed like a vast expansion of inner space, in a different dimension. To me it was like a limitless nothingness, so blinding and bright that it appeared dark, like a massive benevolent black hole, the likes of *Mahankala Shiva*. It was so intense that it became very, very soft, but I felt I was merging into this Divine Being Shiva-Gorakshanath.

As you know, absolute light is total darkness. That is the nature of the light. I know that it is difficult to comprehend this kind of celestial light. That's why we have known that describing it is a futile task, which doesn't even do a shadow of justice to the experience. So when you flash it is as if there is an explosion of a countless supernova in front of your eyes. He just let my awareness, my state of Being, play its role and confirm that it was true. This light is always there when a person is totally dissolved into the "Eternal Now", called God. He is not even an *avatar*, not even a Divine Being. He is beyond that, a total Is-ness of the Zero Naught Zero, Non-being, the Formless One, and more. The more I talk about him, the more of a mess I get into, as the King is beyond all words.

The Shiva-Goraksha-Babaji whose experience I had, is the veritable Lord Shiva himself. He is the Consciousness of the universe. He must not be confused with Babaji Nagaraj, a South Indian saint, or the various yogis going around today with the name of Babaji and or Goraknath.

Due to my past *samskaras*, I have experienced this lofty Presence as Shiva-Goraksha-Babaji. Each time I go deeper into my consciousness, the truth is that I experience him more as the "Non-Being Essentiality," fathomless and incomprehensible.

As a result of this life-transforming experience, I was blessed and empowered by the Great One, and at his behest, my service to humanity crystallized gradually into my mission, which may be stated in three parts.

The first is that it is meditated to the furthering of human awareness by my initiating people into Mahavatar Babaji's *Kriya Yoga*, through *Shaktipat*.

The second part is dedicated to serving humanity as my larger Self by giving my unified Consciousness experience as *Shivapat*. By this experience, people can realize the unity of human Consciousness, to live in peaceful co-existence.

The third part is devoted to making peoples' lives a celebration, by teaching them healing enlightenment techniques through *Pranapat* (breathing through their breath). All these ways and means lead us to Earth-peace through Self-peace.

The receiving of these techniques and the Declaration of Human Rights, after the experience with Shiva-Goraksha-Babaji, left me in a daze. After entering my body gradually, I was no longer in that higher state of *Nirvikalpa Samadhi*. As I came back to my own original state and *sadhana*, the voiceless voice seemed to say to me, "Make your own equation, work out your own *karma*, and be your own enlightenment!"

Who is Babaji?

Babaji, the Divine Being, is the personal aspect and Universal Is-ness of the Absolute Consciousness Shiva. The Divine Babaji, who is your potential true Self, may be realized through persevering *Kriya Yoga* practice. He is not born but comes into manifestation at the beginning of the creation of our three dimensional world.

Although present in the midst of the world of causation, space and time, the Divine Being Shiva-Goraksha-Babaji is not subject to the *karmic* law of cause and effect. He is not bound by any third dimensional laws which govern the mortal body and mind.

In my teaching sincere seekers all over the world, I have become aware of much confusion as to who the Being called Babaji is. Therefore, to clear all doubts and put to rest this perplexity, I have given below who Babaji is, based on my experience and subsequent realization.

- Babaji is *Aja Purush* (meaning unborn). He was never born and therefore can never die. A *Swayambhu*, he Self-manifests from time to time for the salvation of sentient and non sentient existence.

- Babaji Haidakhan who I have personally met has historical evidence to his existance but died a human death, and therefore cannot be the immortal Babaji to whom I am reffering.

- Babaji Nagaraj of south India has no historical evidence but apparently was made to have been born from a human womb and there fore cannot be the immortal (*Aja*) unborn Babaji.

- Babaji-Goraksha Nath also called Shiv Goraksha Babaji has historical references and writings throughout India and is beyond mortal births and deaths. From the night of prehistory even till today His cosmic presence is throbbing in the spiritual aura of humanity.

- Babaji-Goraksha Nath is still alive AND his deathless presence hallows the Himalayan ranges and the spiritual essence of humanity.

He is known by many names but the Being is ever the same. He is also called the Sage of all ages; Shiv-Goraksha, Tryambak Baba, MahaRudra, Maha Avatar The Youth of Sixteen Summers, The Elohim, Yaveh, The Lighting Standing Still. He is the Lightless Light which Lights that Light which Lights the Light of all our Souls, He is the innermost livingness which moves the subtlest life in humanity. Our very being and breath is Babaji in motion and all of us die to live in HIS Immortality.

Babaji-Goraksha Nath (Shiva-Goraksha-Babaji) is the Great Banyan Tree from which sprouted all the *avatars* and prophets from the Ancient of Days. He is called The Great Initiator, who taught the sacred mysteries of God-Realization even to the Sages of the Fire Mist such as Shankaracharya, Dattatreya, Hermes, Christ, Orpheus, Zarathustra, Melkizedek, Buddha, Moses, Maitreya, Agastya Rishi, Lao Tse, Matsyendra Nath, Shams Tabrezee—Prophets, Peers, so on and so forth. The 18 South Indian Siddhas, the 84 North Indian Siddhas, the Nav-Nath (9 Maha Siddhas), are not only His disciples but emanations from this Supreme Being, incomprehensible and great beyond the reckoning of mortals and Celestial Beings.

Compassionate and ever vigilant lest any soul lose its way in the desert sands of materialism; he guards and guides the evolution of our humanity for the whole world-cycle, which for Him is but the wink of an eye. *Babaji* simply means "Revered Father". He goes by many names and yet is called the Nameless One. He is the Visible Invisible Saviour who broods over his infant humanity from eternity to eternity.

> *IF AT ONE MOMENT, TIME AND PLACE*
> *THE SUN-BURST OF A COUNTLESS SUNS OCCURED*
> *THIS WOULD SCARCE SUFFICE TO SHOW THY SHADOW*
> *OH LORD ! WHAT MUST BE THY LIGHT ?*
>
> *-Yogiraj Siddhanath*

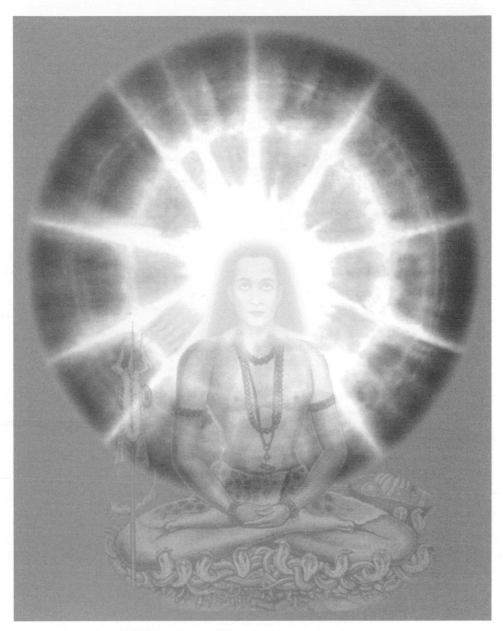

A shadow of one of the actual experiential visions
I was blessed with of Shiv Goraksha Babaji, as
THE LIGHTLESS LIGHT WHICH LIGHTS THAT LIGHT
WHICH LIGHTS THE LIGHT OF ALL OUR SOULS !

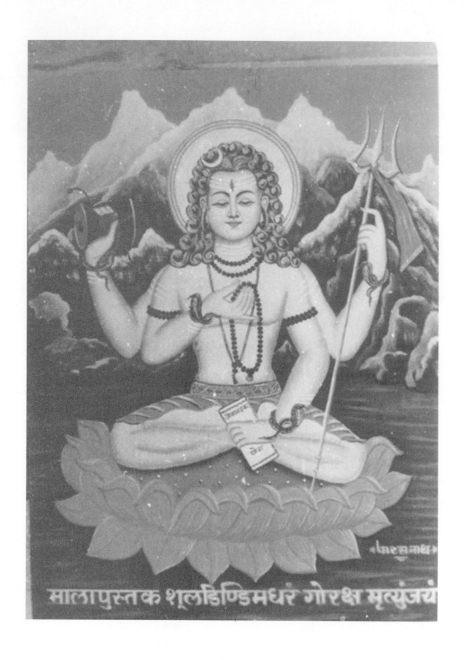

साला पुस्तक शूलडिण्डिमधरं गोरक्ष मृत्युंजयं

Babaji Gorakshanath as Mritunjaya

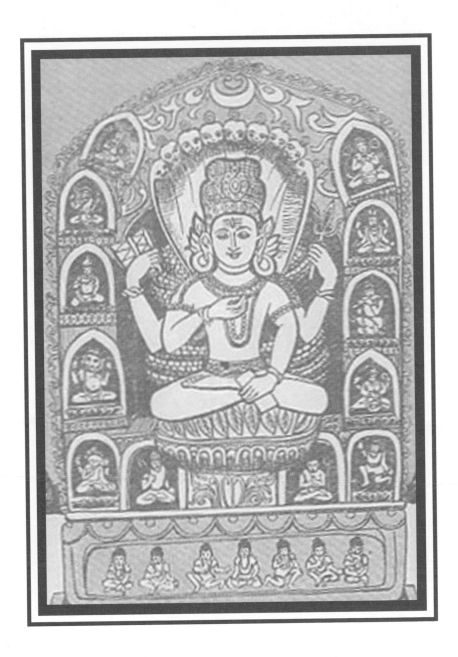

*Babaji Gorakshanath venerated
in Divine form*

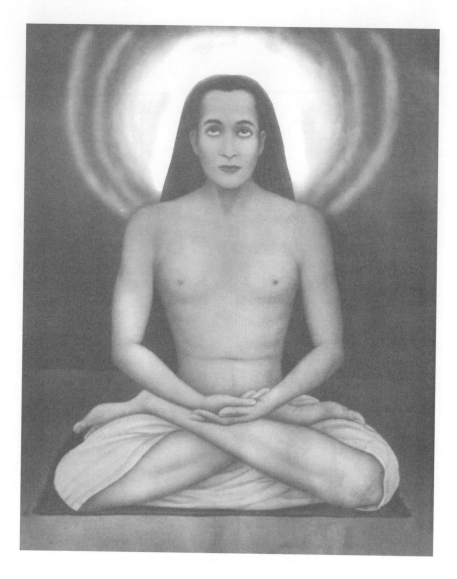

*Original painting of Babaji
guided by Paramhamsa Yogananda*

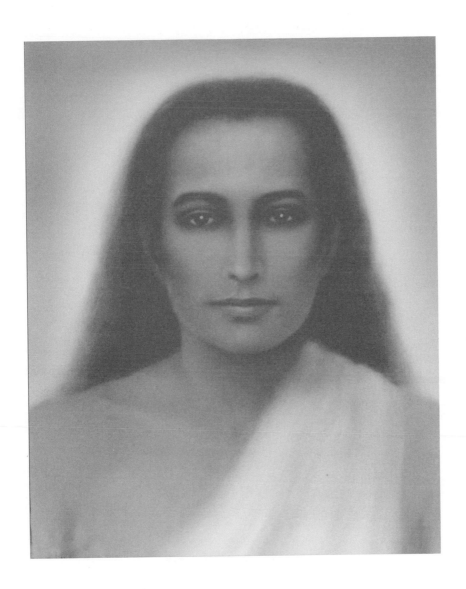

Later contemporary painting of Babaji

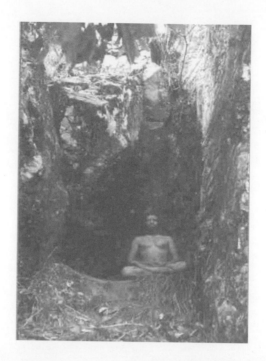

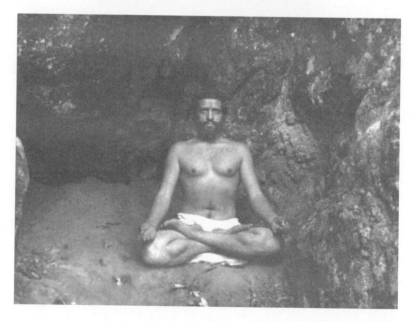

Yogiraj Siddhanath inside the cave of Babaji

CHAPTER 2

EARLY CHILDHOOD

Before my birth, my mother was blessed by the sacred *vibhuti* ash left from the sacred fire ceremony held in honor of Shiva-Goraksha-Babaji. A part of the *vibhuti* ash she ate and a part she kept in her trinket box. During her pregnancy, she was unable to eat much food and lived more on a liquid diet, drinking water mixed with the temple *vibhuti*. She was also blessed by Babaji's great disciple, Guga Chohan, the King of Hiralaya. Every Monday she would go to the temple at Gwalior, my hometown in India. This temple was built by my grandfather after he was blessed with the birth of my father. He dedicated it in honor of these two monumental Beings, Babaji, a Mahavatar[*] and the Chohan King, a great *Siddha* or perfected yogi.

My mother, who had studied astrology, always used to tell me that I would be a yogi, and reminded me that as I was born on the 10th of May in the year 1944, my stars were positioned in such a manner that I was bound to meditate and lead a spiritual life of a householder yogi, like the great *Kriya* Master, Shri Yukteswar. She also had predicted my going to far off lands to teach the timeless science of yoga. This was a blessed birth ordained by Shiva-Goraksha-Babaji, so my mother believed.

My birth was also heralded by great saints and astrologers, who came to visit my grandfather. They spent long hours holding

---

[*] A *Mahavatar* is a *Swayambu* or Self-born manifestation of Lord Shiva, the supreme ascetic and meditative consciousness of the manifested universe and more.

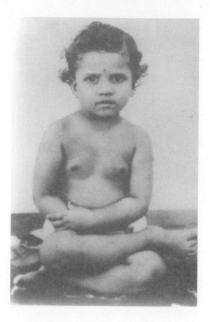

Yogiraj in meditative pose at the age of 3

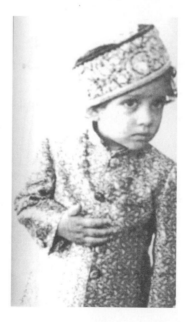

Yogiraj as a child in his princely garb

discourse with him on matters of philosophy, yoga and astrology. They told him that although his grandson would be born in royal pomp and show, ride on elephants and wear jewels around his neck, he would ultimately take to the path of renunciation, would be misunderstood by many and only later in life would his work be appreciated as something of a true contribution to yoga and to the welfare of humankind. He would spread *Sanatana Dharma* (eternal truth) in it's true essence without the religious and ritualistic trappings, which would be beneficial to people around the world.

Being born in the premier aristocratic family of the state of Gwalior, I had ample time to listen to the great epics like the *Ramayana* and *Mahabharata*. These stories are commonly told by parents and elders of the family to children all over India. My mother also told me stories of Gautama the Buddha . I was born in the same month and near to his date of birth. This inspired me greatly along with the stories of Rama and Krishna. Above all I was most deeply influenced by the picture of Lord Shiva in deep meditation. This led me to meditate deeply in the night and in the morning I used to sit with my grandfather to worship the sun by offering oblations with water. But all my *mantras* were taught to me by my father, who had a deep knowledge of chanting and their proper intonation. His deep insight into the *Bhagavad Gita* inspired me to study the sacred and perennial philosophy of India. The *Gita* is a discourse between Lord Krishna, who represents the Spirit, and his disciple *Arjuna*, who represents the Mind. It is one of the most wonderful discourses on the ancient philosophy and the evolution of Human consciousness. My father presented to me my first picture book on the *Gita* at a young age. The second book of the *Gita* he gave me at the age of eighteen and it has been a treasure with me ever since. The sixth chapter is very supportive to my *yogic* practices.

The astrologers and saints of that time had predicted that a boy would be born and that he would be a yogi. I was aware from childhood that I was born from the blessings of Gorakshanath Babaji. However, it was not until later, after investigation, that I found out that the *sanctum sanctorium* of the Kunwar Baba temple was dedicated wholly and solely to Shiva-Gorakshanath-Babaji. Our family *Satguru,* Kunwar Baba called Him *Guru Maharaj*, the same who is the deathless Babaji still alive throughout the ages in the Himalayan ranges; the same Babaji I was to meet at a later time when I matured into a man.

From my earliest months of childhood I was fully aware of my larger Self being housed in a helpless baby body, which was neither able to talk nor to express itself. As a child, everything was a prayer for me because this was the way of our family upbringing. I remember as a child my first effort to stand up on my feet with the support of the sofa. All my spiritual energy rushed up to my third eye as I made this valiant effort to get up onto my own two feet. This was for me my first prayer. It was like a will to do good and to evolve.

As I grew up, my childhood was surrounded with all that I could want. The atmosphere was joyous, and in the big mansion house prosperity and abundance flourished. As the firstborn child of my family, I was pampered and got what I wanted. There are so many things that I do not know how to put a sequence to it. We were one big, large, joyous family with, of course, all the political intrigues going on in smooth harmony simultaneously, as they go on in all aristocratic families. Very amusing it was; from who should wear what jewelry at which function, to which of my aunts should be in the good books of grandfather. They vied for his love and attention by making special meals to take care of him. My father was very interested in horses, so he used to go to Lahore and Peshawar to buy some fine steeds to ride. Although I was young, I realized that it was a part of the game of life.

From the tender age of four I used to sit for long hours in meditation by myself and have visions of Lord Shiva and Krsna in my mind's eye. In the mornings at sunrise, I meditated with my grandfather and always observed what he did. I was very fascinated when he looked at the Sun, taking out his ruby from the golden trinket box; he used to wipe his eyes by rotating the ruby around them. I always used to wonder what this was all about but never got to solve the mystery and he did not care to tell me what he was doing.

While still an infant, my parents temporarily moved to the sacred city of Benares to our family property called *Gai Ghat*, which was located on the banks of the Ganga. The *ghat* had a big stone bull on it, which is why they called it *Gai Ghat*, meaning "the cow bathing *ghat*." Over there was our family temple of Lord *Shiva,* where we all used to worship and meditate. It was very interesting to later find out that alongside our family bathing ground, the monumental *Siddha* called Trailinga Swami used to meditate. All the surrounding *ghats* echoed his name and were hallowed by his Presence. Even before I was born, this great yogi had worked wonders for the spiritual evolution of mankind showing by example, and not by word, what it was to be united with the Divine. He lived on to be over two hundred and fifty years of age. During that period, this renunciate had met the great householder Yogavatar Lahiri Mahasaya, and paid glowing tributes to his spiritual state of realization. The perennial science of Babaji's *Kriya Yoga* was first given to today's world by Lahiri Mahasaya. These are the lofty sages called the "Guardian Wall of Humanity" who protect and nurture the spiritual seed of mankind. Because of them, later saints and yogis evolved into the likeness of their own Divinity. The name of the *ghat*, which this great *Avadhoot Siddha* Trailinga hallowed by his presence, was called Manikarnika bathing *ghat*.

My father, I later came to know, had shifted to Benares because he was to complete some of his higher education at the Benares Hindu University. Dr. Radhakrishnan, who later went on to become the President of the Republic of India, was then the Chancellor. My father, in those days, was given everything he wanted by my grandmother. He made use of a small seaplane to fly over the river Ganges and often used it to transport himself to the Hindu University. But in spite of his academic schedule, he found time to visit the great Yogi Trailinga, whose blessings definitely must have been upon his head. I feel the blessings of the sage must have influenced my spiritual growth as well after he had left his physical abode. Those were great days at our riverside house and *ghat* at Benares. I remember catching the bars of the low window, looking out at the flowing river Ganga with my golden hair blowing in the breeze (which came all over my eyes) wondering why other children's hair was black and mine was gold like a halo of sunshine around my face. I loved to bask in the sun as a baby, even from the age of three, little knowing that later I would initiate a process of Solar meditation and healing called the *Surya*.

Once my parents had left me in the house in Benares and had gone to the main temple of Lord Shiva called Kashi-Vishvanath. They later went to the temple of Hanuman, the monkey god, so I was told by Ramlal Ullu, our family servant in whose care and custody my parents had kept me. "*Ullu*" means owl or idiot. So true to his name, Ramlal left me alone in the courtyard and went into the house to do some work. When he came out, to his utter surprise and dismay, he saw a golden-locked baby of three sitting on the lap and held in the arms of a she-monkey on the roof of the house. That was me! I was feeling quite at home and comfortable with no fear or embarrassment of any sort. Then Ramlal came with milk and *jalebi* (a sweet) to entice the monkey to come down, and thankfully, the monkey quickly responded, leaving me on the terrace. Ramlal then went and retrieved me while heaving a final sigh of relief. When my mother came back she was shocked and furious at the servant for being so careless and later summed it up with "It's all the protection of Shiva and Hanuman."

My grandfather used to take me for a dip in the holy Ganges, which I tended to dread because he would put me underwater a bit too long. I thought to myself that Grandpa has lost his sense of time, and complained to Grandma. The dips in the Ganges and the holding of my breath underwater became less torturous.

At the age of five my grandfather brought me a watch, which stopped after a few days. Thinking it to be dead, I gave it a ceremonial burial in the back yard and decided to set off for the Himalayas. I could take the idea of men dying, but to see a watch die was the final blow to my positive way of thinking. I thought to myself, "This is the last straw. If living things die, it's okay, but when dead things die, I'm through with life." A deep shadow was cast over my heart and I thought I should renounce like the Buddha or something, find ways to eternal peace and not feel so bad about things. So I decided to go to the Himalayas and do intense meditation and ask God what all this dying and stopping was about. I thought he was playing with us, bringing us to birth, only to have us die about eighty years later. So to overcome death and be immortal in God's Eternity became my quest from then on.

That incident took place in the town of Shivpuri. My uncle, who was a good six years older than me, decided to accompany me. As we set out for the Himalayas on foot, we enjoyed the dusty morning on the road in the sunrise while being blissfully ignorant of the direction or the distance to the Himalayas. We had not even the sense to take any money with us as we set out, only a few clothes and belongings, inspired by the tales and stories of great yogis and Divine Beings like Dhruva, Buddha and Prahlad.

Hardly an hour had gone by when hunger started assailing us and our resolve softened. Then to crown it all, my young uncle began to tell me stories of the ferocious tigers in the Himalayas and of the big pythons, which could swallow up a complete man. So with these tales my footsteps slowed down and we decided to get something to eat. The choice before us was either that we go begging for alms, which we had never done, or to see if it was possible to go back home, have lunch, and set out for the Himalayas again. Too tired to go on, we sat down under a tree and closed our eyes in meditation posture like the great yogis of ancient India. I opened one eye occasionally to see whether anyone was looking at us or attracted to us, but no one came nor ever asked. Nobody was impressed by our yogic meditation stance. So after half an hour we gave this up as a bad joke and started trudging home.

We had walked and hitched a bullock cart ride for a good eight to ten miles, and being only five years of age, my little legs were tired. I kicked up the dust as I walked back in the late afternoon heat. Ultimately we reached home. I met my grandfather and told him excitedly that I had made an unsuccessful trip to the Himalayas. Without looking up from his newspaper he told us to go have food. This concluded our first mighty Himalayan expedition. The thought ran across my mind, "What will Shiva-Goraksha-Babaji say of this? I hope I haven't let him down." But by the wonderful comforting sleep I had that night and the guiltless satisfaction I felt the next morning, I knew that I hadn't let him down and that all was well.

At one time, when the Ganges was in spate, my father and a family friend of ours, exercised by swimming across the river. Those young gentlemen also decided to make a champion of me (which I did become later) by throwing me into the Ganges and then catching me like a ball after I fell into the water. It so happened that one day I slipped from their grasp and was lost from them for a moment. With their hearts in their mouths, they frantically searched, and dove under the water to pull me out by one leg.

As I grew up, I carried on with my meditations day after day, sitting long hours with my grandfather, doing my lotus posture and developing my *Om Namah Shivaya japa*. As I evolved and matured internally, it dawned upon me that the delicate breath of life was fraught with many dangers and could break one's journey. So the only way to make it unbreakable was to connect each breath with God. Later my grandfather taught me the *Ham-Sah mantra*, a silent form of asserting that God and I are one. The practice of this *mantra* calmed my mind and proved to be very transformative in nature. Many people also chant a variant of this mantra called *So-Ham*, both of which are silent intonations done with a passive observation of the inhaled and the exhaled breath.*

> *Hamsa Eternal how may we*
> *Being work-bound yet be everfree?*
> *Enlightened action is the key*
> *Which gives that final liberty!*
>
> *Enlightened action doth arise*
> *Within your crystal conscious skies*
> *Experience of the Hamsa Still*
> *Makes you know Divinity's will*

---

*The yogis chant the *Ham-Sah mantra* with every breath. This is also called the *Ajapa Gayatri Mantra*. Another very effective spiritual practice is to mentally chant the sacred syllable *Om* with every inhaled and exhaled breath.

CHAPTER 3

DIVING INTO THE WATERS OF LIFE
Days of Learning and Growing up

My parents decided to curb my wild ways and civilize me by sending me to school, the Lawrence Lovedale Military School at Ooty, a hill station in Southern India. We didn't do much study there, but spent most of our time imitating the body language of the big sergeant and sticking our tongues out as he turned his back on us. He was a hefty man, an old war horse of the British army, red faced, and with big boots. Once it just so happened that as we stuck our tongues out, he turned around and saw us. Being caught in this uncivil act, we were made to run around the china-pen children's playfield holding our belts on top of our heads, sweating it out in our little battle jackets.

It was soon time for study and as I entered kindergarten, I felt like a scholar of some accomplishment, that is, until they demoted me to the lower kindergarten for not being able to read a story of the pancake. I had some difficulty in spelling pancake. In the lower kindergarten all of the kids would sleep. All in all, this was an easier and much more comfortable scenario where I smoothly slid into the sleeping class.

In a moment I was with the sleeping angels of the lower kindergarten. Now this gives you an idea of my state of mind, how I later revolted against the mind and went on to educate people from all walks of life into the "No-Mind State of Expanded Awareness," bereft of thought and devoid of breath. I felt then, as I feel now that it is the ideal way to exist because there is no aging process in the "No-Mind State". A consciousness unfettered by the chains of thoughts can soar

30

to the highest truths of spiritual splendor. Later on I wrote a poem, a part of which I offer to you here:

Mind Transformation

As a leaking vessel never can fill
Waters of Life so pure and still
So distracted mind fails to retain
Wisdom's nectar in its brain

To ease disease of random mind
A remedy suitable we must find
A rhythmic breathing tension free
With absorption the sovereign key

Steady poise the arrow your will
And shoot the fleeting mind to still
The deer of thoughts, hinds & harts
Felled by your concentrated darts

As one by one they die away
Mind opens up to new day
Streams run tranquil willows sway
Here tame and gentle deer do play

Tamed and tuned to natures flow
Mind melts into the opal glow
Which radiates from the soul within
Where Wisdom's mystic fire is King!

During my kindergarten days, there was then an American craze introduced into Indian society called the "chewing gum," which I savored very much. I was given a packet of this gum by one of the senior girls from our sister school, and was chewing it, when our matron, a tall Australian lady, was quick to capture the movement of my mouth and promptly had me spit it out as though I had committed some unpardonable crime.

She then ceremoniously took me to the bench and made me stand up on it in front of all the girls and boys. A new emotion sprung up in me as my ears and face turned red. I felt nobody should watch me when I was not wrong. Later my elementary school friends told me with a scholarly air that this emotion was called embarrassment.

That night after supper, as I went to bed I sat up and meditated with my blanket over my head, lest this also be an unpardonable crime. But nobody checked me and I went into a deep state of awareness. A point of light spread from my Third Eye and bathed my whole body. Said the light, "Whatever you do, meditate always."

Mathematics was never dear to me, and so I was happy to leave this old school, only to be admitted into a new one at the foothills of the Himalayas called Sherwood College in Nanital. This hill station was a very beautiful place with nine lakes, beautiful sylvan surroundings and the snowy mountains like Shiva's laughter to enhance its beauty. I was not told the reason for my change of school. My uncle Jai Singh and my aunt Sanyogita were also transferred to this school along with me. Sanyogita was in the sister school, "All Saints," and my uncle and I were both in Sherwood. This place, to my way of looking at it, was an ideal place to meditate and acquire true knowledge rather than academic knowledge. And so the quest began, my search for the Himalayan yogis. But this was an inward learning sacred to me, that I kept to myself, while around me swirled the routine and clamor of daily life.

Subjects like algebra, math and trigonometry were otherworldly to me. Once I suffered a stroke of genius and I maxed a small trigonometry paper in a weekly test, getting 15 out of 15 marks. The teacher threw a fit at my progress and threatened to throw a party in my honor, which he of course never ever did. If he had, it might have been a different story today. Chemistry was not so good but history was okay. My favorite subjects in school were painting, art, and Divinity (Bible studies), which our missionary teachers taught to us thoroughly. The alpha and omega of Christian thought I absorbed and grasped with great ease. Later at the age of sixteen, I summed it up with the original sin of Adam and Eve relishing the apple at the center of their bodily garden of Eden. This led to the downfall of humanity into procreative sin, then ending with Jesus who was crucified for the redemption of the sins of mankind.

I felt then, as I do now, that this teaching leaves no space for self-grace nor for valiant endeavors formerly made by great souls to achieve salvation. It reminds me of a saying, "Let us have wine, women and laughter, and sermons and soda water the day after." People would then tend to put undue burden on Lord Jesus who they think has already redeemed them, resting satisfied in the false notion that whatever they did, the Messiah would redeem them. This would lead to indolence of the human will. A sacrifice made by another soul—no matter how great—to save all other lesser souls, who had no part in their own salvation or evolution, was to me a very dissatisfying philosophy lacking self-esteem.

The true teachings of Jesus were to love humanity and by sincere self-effort be with God. "Follow me," he said, "and I will make thee a fisher of men." By this he meant that through self-effort enlighten oneself and then teach deserving men to strive for their own salvation. He taught more by example and his meditations and way of life strengthened my belief of his being a great yogi and a true man of God.

Yogic meditation was by far more than a subject to me. It was the Self-same me and I reveled in it and drank it until I was so drunk with my meditations that I often missed the import of academic studies. However, I was still thirsty for a deeper knowledge from the Himalayan yogis—the knowingness of in-depth meditation and an actual experiencing of Divine Ecstasy and *samadhi*, which the scriptures could not afford me. As I grew up, my desire became intense. I told this to no one and those to whom I did tell never understood what it was all about...the Himalayas, the yogis. So at night I kept my meditation constant and steady as I went deeper and deeper. But in the morning times I had to keep myself content with chapel hymns, "The King of Love My Shepherd Is" and "There Is a Green Hill Far Away". As my meditations deepened, my academic studies worsened, since I was no scholar, but meditation with me was a passion. Nevertheless, in our day-to-day trivial 'round the common task, we broke little rules and were checked by the senior house prefects who broke the bigger rules. Our house monitors (called prefects) were by no means perfect. The saying, *"it's human to err, but it's so delightful"* still holds water.

Aside from the Christianization of my mind, which I thoroughly liked, my days of rowdiness, fun, and studies at school flowed on. But in the undercurrents of my mind, there arose a deeper flame to bathe in the lilac lagoons of my consciousness, with the ancient sages and be initiated into the ancient mysteries of yoga, lost in the twilight of history. To drink of the "Waters of Life" from those lagoons of perennial knowledge and as in ancient days, be like those grand *yogis*, the Sons of the Fire Mist, the monumental *Siddhas* who formed the Guardian Wall of Humanity, such was my ambition. But alas! in those younger days, my conduct did not match my ambitions. In my wild ways, I wrongly imagined my progress. As St. Peter so well put it, "Oh Lord, the spirit is willing, but the flesh is weak!" I longed to be like those great Nath Yogis, the colossal Janus-faced transformers who with one face absorb the mighty cosmic currents of the Universe to save humanity from harm's way, and through the other face transmit benevolent radiation to humanity for the spiritual evolution of their Consciousness.

If it had not been for these Masters and *Siddhas*, not only would this world have been a poorer place to live in, but humanity itself would be unable to withstand the stupendous cosmic *Kundalini* surge which would have wiped it off the face of the earth. This is the inconceivable work of the mighty *Siddhas*, the monumental *Avadhoots* and ineffable *Avatarnaths* by whose very breath we live. It is in the aura of these Nameless Ones, far beyond the reckoning of mortal man, that we live and move and have our Being. Special mention must be made of the supreme importance of the "Lightning Standing Still," called the "Visible Invisible Savior of Mankind". He is called the "Great Sacrifice," the "Lightless Light which lights that Light, which lights the Light and all our Souls". He is the head, the heart, the seed and the Soul of undying Knowledge. His aura is spread beyond Eternity. He broods over many infant humanities and shall keep doing so and evolving all Souls into the likeness of his Being. Heaven and Earth shall pass away, but he will be with us to stay. Such is the Great Sacrifice. This is *Shiva-Goraksha Babaji*, "He About Whom Naught May Be Said".

One lazy afternoon, while I was not at all in the mood for studying, we were in the chemistry laboratory and my mind wandered and soared high in the clouds, accompanying the birds, gliding carefree through the vast space. Some boys were serious with their elements, compounds and mixtures, creating queer and rare odors and stinks in the laboratory. My mind was a floating cloud. When the chemistry teacher looked at me, I picked up my test tube and poured one colored chemical into another colored chemical. What I was doing I didn't know, but the reaction was violent and a sudden effervescence occurred letting out a lot of stinking steam. My hands were burned after that as I came to my senses and later realized that I had mixed some hydrochloric acid with some other substance of which I hadn't the faintest idea. Why I was doing all this chemical stuff, I didn't know. Why my parents had sent me to this hell of a laboratory, I didn't know.

I prayed earnestly to Lord Shiva to liberate me from this chemical ordeal. Just then somebody mixed a potion called hydrogen sulfide and, God help us, for only those who know will know the smell of it. I said to myself that since I am a yogi of unperturbed mind let not this laboratory odor ruffle me. So with a stoic face I endured the ordeal, but not for long.

No sooner had I prayed, a messenger came rushing in from the principal's office saying that myself, an American boy called Bobby Myers, and Kenneth Khan, were required immediately. It was to render assistance in a drowning accident at the lake. I rushed headlong out of the laboratory to my dormitory, slipped my swim trunks on, buttoned my trousers fast, and with the other two guys, ran at a steady pace down to the Nanital Lake. Bobby was saying, "Run slow guys, we've gotta preserve our stamina. If the lake is deep, you've got to hold your breath long." "Oh! We'll be given oxygen cylinders for the operation," said Kenneth. I said, "You guys, don't jump to conclusions. You don't even know whether the guy has drowned or is in the process of drowning. Let's just make for it. Anything's better than the obnoxious gas of the chemistry lab."

Pit pat went our feet as we all steadily ran down the hills and made our way towards the lake. On reaching the spot, we found that there was nobody to rescue. Within a trice, the three of us had our clothes off and were ready to dive in with our swim gear. We were told that the mishap had already occurred and a boy from the Birla College had already drowned.

Our school staff and authorities pleaded with some local doctors for oxygen cylinders, so that we could go down and rescue the body, but this was to no avail, as there was a shortage of oxygen cylinders. Nobody knew the depth of the lake on that spot, but it was estimated to be 40 feet. This entailed a risk of all of us bursting our eardrums due to the water pressure or running out of our own capacity to hold our breath and in the bargain of rescuing the drowned boy, drowning ourselves.

So three boats were brought, into which we jumped, one for Bobby, one for me, and one for Ken. So Bobby took the first dive and came back up after about a minute, visibly shaken and disturbed. On asking what the matter was, he said it was a futile task to dive in the lake, as after 20 feet the water resisted his going down and he was compelled to use super propulsion of hands and feet, burning lung oxygen very fast.

I took the second dive. It was deep, dark, green and cold. Suddenly a current of cold water went through my body and abdomen like a spear passing through me. I had no idea how deep I had gone and couldn't see a thing. I used my hands and feet to propel me lower, keeping in mind that I had to save some lung oxygen to enable me to surface again. Then without touching bottom, I turned and swam upward again knowing that if I didn't do it now, I'd not make it to the top. On my upward journey something long and cold slithered by my body and back. Now this really gave me new speed since I obviously thought it to be a big water snake or an eel of sorts.

When I came up and sat in the boat, I saw the hill to the side of the lake filled with a sea of faces. Thousands of people had come to watch and give lip sympathy to the drowned boy as well as us. So this made us feel that perhaps we may drown in the attempt too. Then Bobby said to me, "These guys are giving us rotten sympathy." And I said, "Yes. They make us feel as though we are the sacrificial lambs." Then just at the wrong time, Bobby Myers was having a déjà vu of having been down to the lake and not coming up again. So he scared the hell out of me and he was saying my mom's waiting at home and my father's going to buy me a new mobile bike and all these things. I told him to shut up and not weaken our resolve by these thoughts. "Let's do the best we can, as we are in the thick of it," I said.

In the meanwhile, Kenneth had taken his dive but was not a strong enough swimmer to make much headway. So our principal, or the headmaster, withdrew him from the quest at his own discretion. This time the staff had come and tied a rope around us, gave us a torch in our hands and decided to send us down sitting on a big boulder tied to a rope. I focused my awareness in the *shiva-netra* (third-eye), which was my nature to do. Having polarized my energy there, I drew on my inner strength, and held onto the awareness. As they let me down into the deep green lake, my mind was very strong. I descended to the bottom of the lake and sunk into a mossy substance of two to three feet deep, which I couldn't see, but could amply feel.

All of a sudden in the darkness something brushed my cheek like a hand. I flung the torch, abandoned the stone on which I descended and with full vigor and strength I breast stroked my way towards the surface. My yogic *pranayama* had given me this extra stamina and was sure coming in handy at this moment of crisis. But the surface of the lake never came, and my courage or foolhardiness was not in me as I struggled on. My lungs were filling up and tightening and I had a very temporary flash of a blank out, about a second, then I was back to my senses. Then after what seemed to be forever I surfaced about thirty yards away from the boat, which was there for me, heaved a mighty gulp of oxygen and exhaled all my dead breath out to be born anew. I was sure baptized in the soup of blue green lake by the water god Varuna.

Before I took the next dive I waited for 20 minutes. In the meanwhile a few other expert divers had come to join us and though the body was retrieved later, it was of no avail because his spirit had long departed from his body of clay.

That night, as I lay in my bed wide awake, the truth occurred to me, that here was this dead body who didn't even try to drown. He had another life saver by his side and he still drowned. He didn't try to die, but he died. Here we were, stretching our luck to the uttermost, by a possibility of drowning, with no oxygen cylinders, and yet we were saved. Such is destiny. Life is truly destiny by one's own past *karma*, the laws of which human beings cannot fathom, but they must dig deep the well of their consciousness to realize the ultimate Truths. This event later led me to compose a poem on *karma*, the underlying justice meted out to every being due to the present reactions to their past actions.

I here offer to you, to read, mark and to inwardly digest a few verses from my poem taken from the book, "Dew-drops of the Soul".

Karma

To reap what you have sown
Is God's Mathematical Law
All wrongs must be redressed indeed,
This fact it has no flaw.

All rights are rewarded
In proportion and no more.
To each one is meted out
His exact and proper score.

This unbribable Judge we people,
Call "The Karmic Law".
The supervisor of the Fates
Of our worldly see-saw.

Who justly balances the ups
And downs of lives of man
Fitting the jigsaw of our fates
As we ourselves had planned.

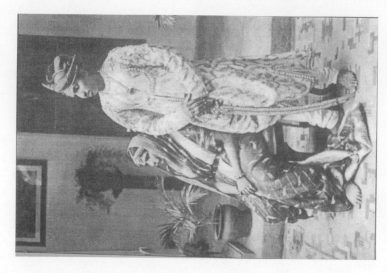

Shri Krishnarao & Sou Snehalata Raje Sitoleh
Father and Mother of Yogiraj

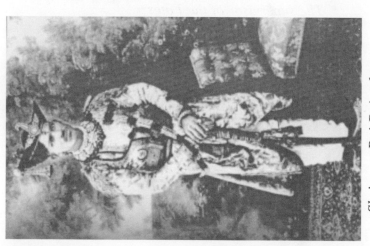

Shrimant Raj Rajendra
Malojirao Sitoleh Raja Deshmukh, Pune
Grandfather of Yogiraj

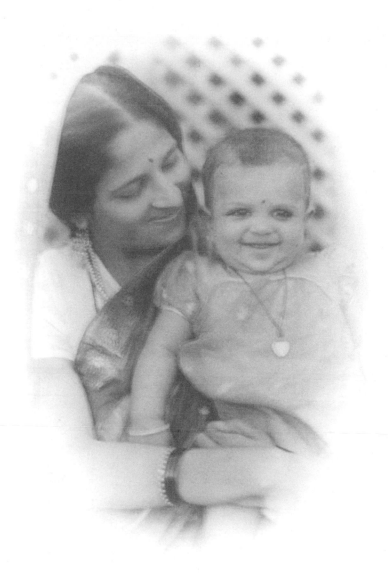

Yogiraj as a baby in the arms of his mother

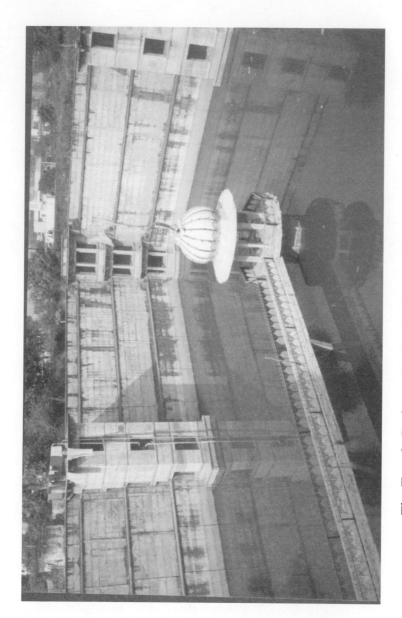

The Temple Bath at Gwalior built in honor of Guru Guganath by Yogiraj's grandfather on the occassion of his son's birth

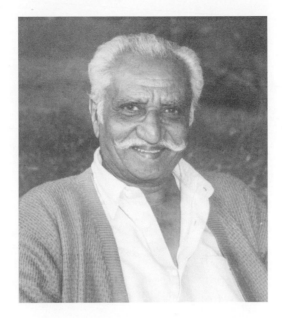

Father of Yogiraj Krishnarao Sitoleh

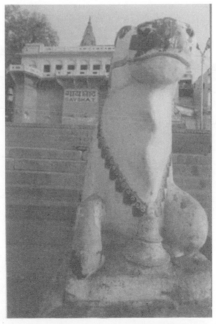

Gai Ghat, the Sitoleh ancestral temple, on the banks of the Ganges in the holy city Varanasi (Benares)

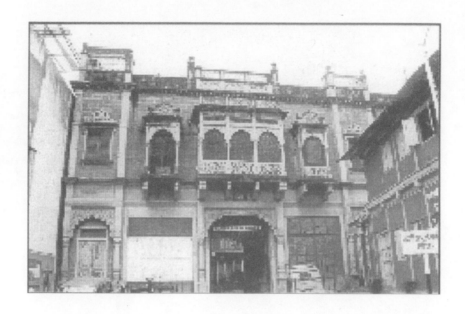

Gurunath's ancestral home in Pune

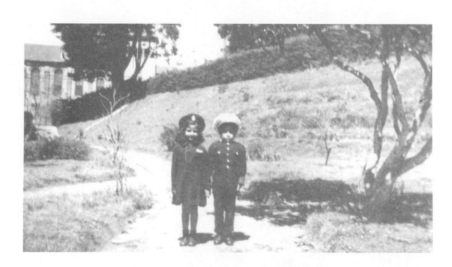

Yogiraj at Lawrence Lovedale Military School
with young aunt Sanyogita after Sunday Chapel Mass

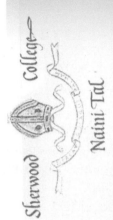

Sherwood College

Naini Tal

This Certificate is awarded to
SIDHOJI RAO SHITOLE
in recognition of his courage
in descending repeatedly to
the bottom of the Naini Tal
lake, on 18 September 1962, in
depths of thirty to forty feet,
to render assistance in a
drowning accident. ✧✧✧✧✧

R. C. ...
Principal

Yogiraj's Certificate of Valor

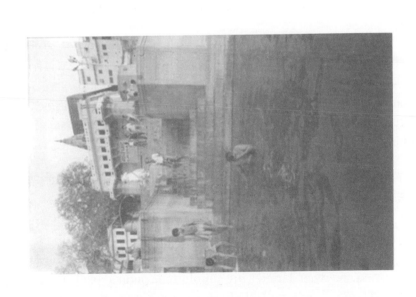

Bathing scene at Gai Ghat, Varanasi

CHAPTER 4

PREPARING THE INNER MASTER
A Turning Point: Babaji Gives a Sign

My education at Fergusson College in Pune was completed in 1967. I then set about finding a job in some of the industrial companies in Pune. Because of my father's connections, I was interviewed and employed in a German factory called Backau Wolf. The factory specialized in manufacturing equipment for sugar factories.

So I settled down to work in the purchase department of the company. My body was at the desk, but my heart traveled far away to the Himalayas, and the spiritual abodes of the Indian saints and yogis.

Many a time I was found lacking in my ability to cope with the work I was assigned. So there I was, a purchasing officer in charge of the purchase of centrifugal machinery parts. I tried to adjust as best I could, but often found myself meditating at my office desk instead of working.

One day my senior officer, Mr. Shweres came to me, and told me that there was an urgent requirement for thirteen "flowell solenoid" valves. Our clients were coming in two days and I was told to get the thirteen valves. So I began contacting and phoning all our suppliers one by one. There was clearly a non-availability of these valves. I was worried and when I tried a big supplier, he phoned back and told me he had none. I requested him to please look in the warehouse and recheck. He did and told me there were no "flowell solenoid" valves.

The next day, I went to the office, and in spite of trying to work, I went into a deep meditation. I prayed earnestly, "Oh Lord, since I am in communion with you, I have little time to search for the valves. Could you please help me just a little bit? Get them for me oh Lord." Other people in the office were amused at my style of office work. When I came out of my state of meditation, the telephone rang, and I went and picked up the phone - it was the big supplier I had phoned the day before. He said that he had found the "flowell" valves in the morning. I found this to be quite uncanny. So I asked, "How many?" He replied that there were only thirteen in stock. This incident had an astounding effect on me, and an overwhelming love for the Divine welled up.

I thought to myself, "If the Divine had answered such a small prayer for me, how infinite must be his love? What am I doing serving a sugar company, when I should be washing the feet of the Lord with the nectar of my heart.?" This was the turning point in my life. I left the company job to serve my beloved, the Divine. So I endeavor to serve humanity, to serve Shiva-Babaji to this day. To be in communion with him who is in all.

The Inner Master Unfolds

I then set out for the ancient city of Vrideshwar where Lord Shiva initiated the Nath Yogis into the ancient mysteries of the universe. A little distance away from this town is a sacred shrine of the great Matsyendranath where people pray and get their wishes fulfilled even to this day. Arriving in the city, riding a bullock cart, I became overwhelmed with the atmosphere of freedom and gave all my belongings to the needy and the children in the village.

My mind was still as in *unmani avasta* and nothing seemed to really matter except communion with the Divine. My mind was as a tranquil lake, free of the ripples of any kind of thoughts. This stillness experience I remember having since childhood, but a new phenomena arose within me making me identify more and more with my Conscious

Seer and less with my mind.

As my days of meditation in Vrideshwar went by, I was more easily able to raise my consciousness up and out of my mind's lake to identify with my Supra-conscious Seer, my vaster Divine Self. But at times, from the depths of my mind's lake, bubbled up some past life memory impressions and mental images, which I dissolved by the practice of my yoga. I realized these experiences of the unfolding of my consciosness to be the result of my past life's evolutionary meditation and *tapa*.

Not only was this identity transition from the phenomenal mind to the nomenal Consciousness happening more often, but I also found myself being able to transfer both my mind energy and Conscious awareness to others, and people began to experience my peace and bliss. By the grace of Babaji-Gorakshanath my Self became able to teach not only with words, but also by giving others an actual experience. The experience I gave to others was of my state of mind, which was of a healing nature. Clearly my inner Master, due to my past life *samskars*, was unfolding and being prepared to be a servant of humanity and spread the good work of the evolution of human consciousness. My natural inclination is to meditate on pure Consciousness and aspire for the states of *samadhi*. The merging of my individual consciousness into the infinite Consciousness is my path of Yoga. But meditation with form and visions of the Divine have their proper place too.

The Coming of the Siddhis and their Rejection

I slept at the Rama temple at night. I could hear Shiva's bull going into Shiva's temple nearby. After I visited Udaipur at a later date, my family genealogy and my past life connections to my present life became very clear to me; I was put in the Rama temple because he is my ancestor, I belong to his lineage. We are *Suryavanshis*, meaning descendents from the Sun-god (*Surya*). Rama was forty-seventh in descent from Ikshavaku of the solar dynasty. This whole genealogy - this whole lineage is recorded right up to our present family. That is why I was in the Rama temple to meditate and to worship.

As I sat in the temple meditating, people started coming and visiting me. Village women came with their children and laid them before me. I didn't know what they were saying or why they were laying them before me because I was focused on another world. These people came from yet another world. Since I used to meditate with palms up, some people used to throw a cent or two in my hand, as if I were a mendicant or beggar by the road. I thought this was a good way to humble my ego. The Sitolehs of Sisodias claim to be princes of certain places, and now they are getting a cent, sometimes even a coconut! That's good survival. But I didn't bother about this because I was not in myself. I was only aware of these offerings when I returned to normal consciousness.

Then a boy called Dashrath came and I said, "Okay Dashrath, what do you want?" He said, "My head hurts and I always have pain on the right side of my head and right side of my body." I said, "Okay, come here." When he came close I gave him one tight slap on the right side of his face. My healing processes are different! He literally fell down. The next morning he came with a big glass of milk. I said, "Why have you got this?" He told me, "After you slapped me, the pain never came back again. I am totally cured." So I asked, "Now what do you want?" He said," Give me something." I closed my empty fist. When I opened my hand, there were pomegranate seeds in it, so I gave him these seeds. He said, "Now can you give me a mango?" I said, "Okay, you will have a mango. I will not produce it but your stomach will feel the mango juice pouring in. You'll feel it flowing down into your stomach, and when you belch, the whole room will be filled with the aroma of mango." So he did experience that. And he said, "Yes, I was drinking mango juice, got the whole flavor of mango and then burped! When I was drinking I could feel it, when I burped I could smell my own burp, it was so fragrant."

So these *siddhis* started coming to me. When I did spontaneously produce things with a few people I thought, "No, this is not my path. This is a deviation. These are the powers of the Soul. I don't mind using healing powers, and I don't mind bringing ectoplasmic material from the astral world into the physical world. But the sanction must come from the top. It must come from Shiva-Goraksha-Babaji."

Unless directed from above, the using of these supernatural powers for selfish or healing purposes deludes the yogi from the true path of Self-Realization. Although the using of the siddhis for materail pofits temporarily satisfies one's ego and makes one feel great, but when compared with the ecstasy of God communion is like comparing pieces of glass with true diamonds. No serious yogi on the path would like to trade the bliss of divine communion for transient siddhis. It is unwise to fritter away the energy of one's soul to avail oneself of the tinsel wealth of an evancescent world.

Then I went on my way and I knew that I had to move inwards. As I intensified my meditations and *pranayama,* my diet became almost negligible. My body felt light as a feather and the boundaries of my inhibited mind melted and became the boundless ocean of consciousness, disregarding all other worldly wants. I strove and stretched my yogic practices to the limits and as I dove deep into the depths of my knowingness, I became aware of the continuity of this life's meditation from my past life. In spite of myself my meditations became my natural Self.

During my spaces of solitude, all spiritual experiences stopped for a few days. I did not give much importance to experiences over that of my *samadhi* or my *unmani avastas.* But I was young, and going through a stagnant and dry phase of my *sadhana* and all spiritual progress seemed to stand still. While praying to Lord Shiva, I yearned to merge into him by the effortless effort (that is what *shramana* means and Shiva is the Supreme *Shramana* and ultimate ascetic, without whose sacrifice the Creation would not spiritually evolve). Reaching for the goal of God contact day in and day out, I made it my life's purpose to find the Divine in this life, even if it meant laying my life on the line. "This is easier said than done," I said to myself. But then I reprimanded myself for the feeble after-thought.

Experience of Goddess Durga while Washing Clothes

I'd heard of a small village nearby where there was a holy shrine to Lord Datta. Before I went to it, I thought I should sit and take care of my clothes. It was late afternoon, two or three o'clock, but I couldn't wash my clothes because I'd never washed clothes before. I only had two sets of clothes that were unstitched garments, each having one bottom and one top. When I wore one set, I washed the other. While I was trying to wash one of my loin cloths, figuring out if I should hammer it, I thought, "It's quite thin and if it tears I shall have no clothes to wear." Just then, a lady came along who was about 60 to 65 years old. "Okay," I said to myself, "I'll learn from this lady how she tackles this thing." She was a fair skinned lady, with a big red *tikka* on her forehead, and white *sari* with a saffron border.

"Do you want those clothes washed?" She asked. I answered enthusiastically, "Yes, yes, yes. Can you teach me?" She didn't answer my request but said, "Give them to me," so I did. As she washed them, I was just looking at her and at once became a small child again. Whenever I look at, or get an experience of the Mother, in the Mother Form—not in the *shakti* form which is different—I become a child again and I was admiring her. Within no time she had washed the clothes and put them out to dry. She made it look so easy but I couldn't understand how she had done the whole thing. She said, "Just do it, put the clothes in the water and raise them." Then she asked, "You have never washed clothes before? You seem to be from a good family and have not had the need to do this washing."

I said, "No, I've never washed my clothes before." So she started to laugh and I was totally lost in admiration. I just stared at her. I don't know exactly what I admired in her, but there was the motherhood, and something divine about her. It didn't strike me who she was. After that she said, "Okay son, I'm going now". I said, "Thank you very much." I kept looking at her, something was wrong. Was I missing the point?

51

She walked to a building behind which the road turned to the left and then went on to the village of Pathardi, quite a long road. As she turned the corner, I got up and ran, exclaiming, "Oh, God! Let me grab her feet! This is the Mother. She is the Goddess. This is Durga!" I knew because I had developed the sight that whenever a holy person leaves a spot, an image of the Goddess comes, or the image of Shiva comes, or the image of Jesus comes. Seeing through the camouflage of these divine beings who test me, I am able to tell who they are. That is why they are very cautious about giving me a vision or *darshan*. When they give it to ordinary persons, they don't know, but I have developed the second sight, often called the *shiva-netra* or "eye of Shiva."

As soon as I saw that, I ran to touch her feet and to get her blessings. I ran to the corner of the *ashram* building but as soon as I turned around it, I saw there were no trees, no houses, nothing to camouflage her, just a gentle, different sort of atmosphere which was left lingering there. She had gone, leaving her spiritual aura there. Even if I had touched her, I might have passed out because her electromagnetic aura was so high, but that depends upon her grace. However, it was a very clear and definite vision of Durga in the Mother form, which I had near the village of Vrideswar. I'll never forget it. The sight of her is very specific because she doesn't always come. She came then, so why is she not coming now? It has been a long time. Usually, the more I pray to Lord Shiva, the more Mother comes to me, not Lord Shiva. My *Ishta Devata* is Shiva, but surprisingly visions or *darshans* I have had are of the Divine Mother because of her loving heart. The Mother's heart encouraged me on to the path of Shiva as the formless Universal Consciousness.

After that, the day was spent in a very blissful state. I was easily able to slip into my state of meditation and *samadhi*. Oblivious to the outer world, I had nothing to own, nothing to gain, and nothing to lose. There were no parents, no father, no mother, nothing. There was just me, my Self and the Not-I. My ego self was oblivious as I was reveling in this inner peace, while the body was being buffeted by the elements outside.

My poem comes to mind here of my state.

Where in sylvan bowers I sat
Not in this world nor in that
Just in the joy of Selfing mirth
The odor of the fragrant earth.

Experience with Saint Zanayabai

On another occasion, I went down to the temple and took the *darshan* of Lord Shiva. Around the temple is a courtyard, and in the courtyard were little shops and a very small tea stall. I met all the people there, and an old lady offered me some tea. "Baba will you take some tea?" I replied, "Yes, I'll take some tea." Another fellow came and asked, "Would you like a *beedi*?" The *beedi* is a rolled up dry tobacco leaf. I decided I may as well smoke a *beedi* because it's a good thing to have one. So my lunch was one *beedi* and one cup of tea. I had not eaten for over a week and so the problem of eating had ceased. Only for the first, second, and third day is one troubled. On the latter part of the third day you start normalizing, so no hunger prevailed, no sense of wanting to eat anything. There was no loss of energy, or lack of it either. I was quite okay, quite full of energy. My body felt light as a feather. I felt as though my feet were not touching the ground—it was very good. I had crossed over to the other side. Although this is not advised for everyone, anybody with the right attitude and fitness may undertake a purification fast.

After tea I went to another *dharamsala*, a place where pilgrims come and stay. I went into the *dharamsala* and a very peculiar thing happened. A girl entered who was possessed. I had been sitting there for a while engaged in my daily activities. In my spare time after meditation, I would sit at the camp fire in the evening with the village people, hear their stories, then go to the *dharamsala*, make new acquaintances, and use the night for meditation. The day was spent learning the culture and the pulse of the people there.

The son of the local *pujari*, a very arrogant boy, tried to put water on the possessed girl. Then he said, "Oh it's a bad spirit," and tried to beat her with sticks and a jute slipper, but the spirit didn't go out. Then the possessed girl calmly asked the bald-shaven *pujari* boy, "Have you finished with your monkey tricks?"

"Now," I thought to myself, "this girl is not possessed by an evil spirit. This is something of a more exalted nature." Then the girl said, "Okay. I'm going to make *chapatties* for you all." She made the *chapatties* (unleavened Indian bread) in that state of trance. She kept her hand on the *tava* (frying pan), and then her hand was on the fire, where the *chapatti* was cooking. The *pujari* boy took her hand down and told her that it was not the way to cook. She replied, "I will not listen to you." Then she told the *pujari's* son, who was posing as a great exorcist and spiritual master, that she would not listen to him, but would listen to this yogi (meaning me). "The yogi knows who I am and he will tell you who I am." But I replied, "I don't know who you are. I have just arrived." However she insisted that I tell. She hissed angrily at the *pujari* boy, who fainted. Just imagine, the spirit being who is being exorcised, exorcises the *pujari*. I exclaimed, "Wait, now what's going on here? What are you doing?" Then I meditated and saw Saint Zanayabai, the Maharashtran saint who had pleased Krishna so much that he used to fill up a water pot and bring it to her. The saint did *pranaam* to me as I did to her. She said, "You don't know who you are, but I know who you are." So I said, "Tell me who I am." She answered, "That I won't do. This is not the time. It is for you yourself by your power to know who you are. Also, you are being falsely modest."

Then Zanayabai spoke, "Can you help me to move out of this body? This dear soul needed help so I gave her some nerve energy. She had nervous disorder, and so I came into her body to fill up the gap to make the circulation of the nerves' energy flow. Now my work has been completed, so just say the *mantra* and let me go." I chanted the *mantra*, threw water on her and the spirit left. This was an exceptional experience in the exorcising, not of bad spirits, but rather the freeing of good spirits by the power of *mantra* when they themselves are helpless to get out of the body. This was a good spirit. When the *pujari* became conscious he said, "What happened? I was trying to exorcise." The other people told him he hadn't done it but that the *yogi* had done it. This was one experience which was very beneficial to all of us; to myself (because it added to my knowledge), to the girl (because it cured her nervous disorder), and to the *pujari* boy, as it humbled his false pride.

Spiritual Contest with the Yogini Velsa

There was a wedding that I had been asked to attend, to bless the couple. I told the people that I was not interested after my last experience at a wedding, during which I had to cast out evil spirits. Instead, I went and sat in a little temple, which happened to be the temple of a goddess called Velsa. She was a goddess *yogini*, or *jogan shakti* as we yogis call it. I went in and entered into a state of trance. Ablaze in my trance, I reached out to touch her feet and to take her blessing but the words, "don't do that!" came from her.

I asked, "What's wrong with you? Is there something wrong?" She replied, "There's nothing wrong with me. I cannot have a yogi touch my feet, because I'm a *yogini* myself." I asked, "What are you saying?" Again she said, "You cannot touch my feet. You can touch Gorakshanath's feet and Yukteswar's feet." I then asked of her, "Okay, but can I meditate here?" She answered, "Of course. As a matter of fact, you are meant to meditate here, to get some message."

As soon as I sat down to meditate, a beautiful aroma started coming, and beautiful, soft music started flowing. The *yogini* came before me smiling and offered me fruits. I said, "Look, what are you doing? I am a yogi, a *tapasvi*. Why are you offering me fruits? I haven't had food for almost 21 days now." She said, "You can eat this." I said, "Whether I have it *astrally*, or I have it physically, it's the same. Now, I'm at a stage where I can control it *astrally*, physically, mentally. So don't spoil my *sadhana*, I ask you."

After some time, a vision of a marriage procession flowed before my eyes, quite beautiful, with a band and all. During this vision, the intensity of spirit of this *yogini*, the spiritual energy was coming and garlanding me, and I said, "Wait a minute! I'm not married. I don't intend to get married. So what are you doing?" She said, "No, no. You are to get married. I am the spiritual energy of the girl who is destined to marry you." At that, I thought, "If this happens one more time, here goes." Again the procession came, so I chanted and I threw a *mantra* missile at her feet. She exclaimed, "What are you doing? Are you attacking me with a missile?"

The astral warfare I had with this Velsa goddess, this *yogini*, was a very unique occurence. You could see the missiles going as photons of light, cylindrical missiles. I formed the *mantra* and said, "*Om, Phat! Swaha!*" But I didn't fire the missiles with the intention of destroying the entity in front of me, just to knock her senseless. So, in this way I had begun a missile battle with this *jogan shakti*. This was the first and last time in my life that I had an exchange on a minor scale like Gorakshanath and Matsyendranath had. I was using *astra vidya* (where sound is used as a missile). She used the same technique to ward off my attack and retaliate, but neither of us did it at a lethal level, only at a level of deterrence.

I told her, "I don't want you to upset my *sadhana* here, coming with garlands to me. When I think of Sri Yukteswar and Gorakshanath, I don't want you coming in the middle with your beautiful face and trying to garland me. If I focus totally on the face, on family life, on sex, on creating spiritual children, then I leave my *sadhana*." So she told me, "That is what your *karma* should be. You have to get in unity with me, for I am filled with the *yogini shakti*. We have to evolve yogicly, for I have certain work which I have to fulfill towards you; to look after you, so that you can complete your *sadhana* and take the great step forward in this life. If you do this alone and there is nobody to feed you, nobody to look after you, then you will not be able to focus 100 percent on your *sadhana*. Therefore, that is my work. You have to fulfill your *karma* towards me. I have to fulfill my *karma* towards you. It is an equal give and take." I thought this to be quite a win-win situation, but refused to accept what she said.

Velsa proclaimed, "I am the *shakti* who is going to be your wife. I am Renuka. So you are destined to be married and lead a householder's life as per the directions of Sri Yukteswar and Babaji." I replied, "This makes no sense to me. I have no such desire in my mind. If you approach me again, I am going to fire this missile *mantra*." Then, she took her missile and fired it straight at me. It hit me and I was quite dazed because I was so strong in my *sadhana* and did not expect it to even hit me. Then, I took another one, chanted, and flung it at her. It hit her, and she dispersed into a light while she repeated "*Om Namo Shivaya*", and then returned again. This battle is called *astra* and it went on for an hour and a half.

I continued trying to meditate when she said, "I am the *shakti*, the power and the energy who is in your wife, in Tanjavar." I asked, "Then tell me who I will marry." She said, "You will marry a princess." I said, "Which princess? What is her name?" She answered, "Just now it is formative. I am not a supreme power, but I am the daughter of Sri Yukteswar and also a child of Gorakshanath. So do not be too proud of yourself, yogi, that you are the only child." I replied, "I am not being proud. You are coming and trying to garland me and indicating that I am getting married. I am on a path of intense *sadhana*. Since I am very focused, it would be dangerous if a thought of a woman or girl, a *shakti*, came to mind, as this would distract me." She responded, "That is not the case; this is not true, rather it will enhance your *sadhana*. When you go to ashrams in the future, this *shakti*, which I am, the *shakti* of Renuka will look after you." So I said, "Okay, okay, let's get to the point."

Automatically I had started speaking to her as if she were an equal. It was on a one-to-one basis, except she had a temple in which to stay and I had none. I had the sky as my roof. She said, "The girl shall be from the Bhonsle family, I do not know which." So I asked her, "I want to test you. If I see any girl on the 19th of June—the day of the resurrection of Sri Yukteswar—I will marry that girl and I will know that you are telling the truth." She said, "Okay, done. That is how it will be." And this was the debate with the spirit of Shivangini. This *shakti* was later to be manifest as the *shakti* of my wife, named Shivangini, or Rajkunvar as she was called before her wedding.

On my departure, I was about to do *pranam* but she said, "No, no *pranam* to one another." So I began to leave when she said, "IT'S very difficult to convince a stubborn yogi like you, for your mind is very focused, set like a spear on Sri Yukteswar and Gorakshanath. With that, you are torturing me because with every missile you hurl, you are hurting me."

You see, in India, virgin women, called *kanyas*, have tremendous inborn power. They don't have to do *sadhana* or meditation like we yogis have to. They have that inner *sadbhava* (female energy). But they cannot make the final goal unless it is amalgamated or fused with the male energy. This they could do by remaining celibate and doing it within their *chakras* and their *kundalini*, or they can get married and get to the same goal. It is easier and much faster to get married than to do it alone. It has all to do with divine alchemy and human evolution. The evolution of consciousness is intricately woven with alchemy—the mind, the breath, thought, the vital fluid.

As time passed, I forgot all about my challenge regarding the 19th of June. But sure enough, later on, my parents made an appointment to see a girl. As the nineteenth began coming close, my mother said, "Oh, there is a very nice girl to meet. She is from Tanjavar. She is from the Bhonsles of Tanjavar, related to the King Shivaji's family."

I said, "Look, *Aie* (Mother), I am not interested in all this stuff. I am interested in my *sadhana* and I left my job also. I don't want to get into this stuff because once you get a wife, then you buy her all sorts of *saris* and clothes and you have to get a job all over again to earn money. Then you have children and then worry about education for children, and it carries on and on." She responded, "No, no, this will not carry on. You can always be sensible in marriage. You need not have many children. You can have two." She was very strong about this, and so I just said, "Okay, but don't be disappointed if I say no. It's very difficult. I am not going to get married because I am very engrossed in my meditation." She said, "fine, we will leave it to destiny and to God."

She departed by car on June 18th and went to Bombay to see the girl. So I thought, "Thank God, this is not it." But I did begin to get suspicious because it was so close to June 19. I wondered, "Is this a trick being played on me," and went into the Yukteswar temple to ask what was going on. En route, my parents' car broke down and she had to stop overnight. So it was that my mother met the girl, and put the *tikka* (mark of blessing) on her head on June 19th. When my parents came back, they told me what had happened. Later that very day, without seeing the girl, I said yes to the proposal and that is how I got married a year later. It was like marrying a *yogini*, a *jogan shakti*, from the temple of Renuka Velsa. How powerful and gracious this *shakti* is in the form of Shivangini. This will be seen when she gets through with all the family work and gets into meditation. The *shakti* will then be in its full force. This was an extremely personal and very, very powerfully interesting episode in my life. Sure enough, later it became the main inspiration for my mother center *ashram* in India and my tours abroad.

After the marriage, I used to tell everyone that I would have a son who would be born on a Thursday, and that he would be a great artist. Shivangani used to say, "Are you mad? You are going and telling this to everyone. Suppose he is born on Friday? We don't even have a child, we don't even know." I said, "No, no, no. I just feel he will be a male child and he will be born on Thursday and we will call him Shivraj." She said, "Enough of this. Don't overdo it. There is no child!" As it came to pass, the child was born on Thursday. It was a male child and we had already given him his name Shivraj.

Scorpion Sting

As I laid down to sleep one afternoon, on the bare earth under a tree, wearing just a *lungi* cloth, something came and stung me. My whole body dispersed into sparks of light. Since I was in a healthy state of body and mind, my whole being responded to the sting. My consciousness sailed out of my body. Internally I was fully aware that this was a *karmic* settling of scores.

And then I saw a big scorpion walking away. I asked, "Hey, what was the necessity to do that?" It turned around and looked at me, and I could literally see it smiling. I thought I must have gone mad—gotten withdrawal symptoms, was going out of my mind. Out of my mind I definitely was. I was in God's mind—so I let it go. I said, "Okay, okay, go. Take your bite. I can take your bite…after all, aren't we all aspiring to be Buddha, to be Jesus? Aren't we aspiring to be Gorakshanath? Go scorpion, go enjoy yourself. If you feel like stinging or biting, do it on the bark of a tree or something." He seemed to listen to me, and he smiled and went away. It's quite hazy when I think now of the tail of the scorpion. It's quite a deadly weapon.

I used to be very good at the scorpion *asana*. When I was young I used to do this *asana* and reflected in my pain. I would touch the soles of my feet to the top of my head. This was my favorite *asana*. The scorpion had stung me on my back. I felt the heavy feeling and tingling sensation of the poison gradually spreading through my body. I took my hand and hit myself forcibly on my back! Then, to my surprise the effect reversed and the tingling sensation receded to a point and the scorpion bite disappeared. I had acquired the *siddhi* of healing, but made up my mind not to use it for myself in the future, as far as I could help it.

That was when I knew I had received healing powers, which I use now in a very sensitive and subtle way. But you must properly let people know that it is for their service that this is being done. They are individuals while I'm not; as I efface myself at the time of transmission and know it is *Shakti*, the universal life-force, that is doing it. And yet, people must be aware that this is not some entry into medium-ship. That is the danger. Truly it is the higher Self, the universal life-force, which is doing the healing, the spiritual transmission as the I-ness stands aside. That was the first indication that I had received these powers.

After that scorpion bite, I stayed a few more days, and soon a month was over. I had managed to do this without any food or any financial assistance whatsoever. I had gone without food for over a month. It was wonderful and my body was feeling fresh and weightless. The juices I drank, made my mind as clear as crystal and I was aglow. I reached my states of trance, and had all the experiences that I was supposed to have. It was a wonderful stay.

I had all those spiritual experiences because I totally relied on the Divine. I had totally surrendered to him—we call this *Ishvar Pranidhan*; not to accept anything, not to want anything, but simply to leave it in the hands of the Divine, for he knows best what is good for you. There was no sense of hunger, no fear, no pain. The calling was that I should go back and continue my meditation and *sadhana* at home. There was no money! I'd distributed my money amongst the village people, flinging it to the village boys when I came to the village in a bullock cart.

I had a precognition one month before I left home, so I said, "Okay, if I have to walk, I'll walk it to Pune, for at any case, it's a do or die situation." I had no doubt it would be very easy for me to get back home. I was not functioning through my mind, but only through a purity of heart, which required no thinking, but only knew what it was doing. And I knew that as soon as I was out of the village a car would come. I would sit in the car and go to Pune. I knew that. One month later, I stepped out and walked not even two hundred yards. A car came from behind me and someone said, "Yogi *Maharaj*, you are walking in the dust. Can we give you a lift?" I said, "I'm going to Pune. If there's a place for me, it's okay, otherwise I'll carry on." With this lift, I went back home and met my mother and my father.

This is the long and short of the experience at Vrideshwar. I went into various states. The state of *samadhi* that I entered was very experiential there. At first my states were spontaneous and not at my own will. Only later did I go into my *avastas* at will. It was not a sudden jerk but a gradual "happening" into more profound, deeper, and heightened states of awareness. Thus I went from these states of awareness progressively into the state of *samadhi*. These were all recapitulations of my past life.

Importance of Guidance in Yoga

So the days of meditation, devotion and service to people carried on year after year. The guidance from great masters like Gagangiri Maharaj, Swami Satyanandagiri, Hariharananda, Shiva Bal Yogiri, Neemkaroli Baba, and divine Anandamayima helped me fortify my Self in my meditations and *avastas*. The light of my *Atma Guru* kept pouring intermittently into my consciousness.

The *Shramanic* teachings of the Nath Yogis led me to a still-mind awareness by the *Amanaska Yoga* of Gorakshanath of which *Hamsa Yoga* teachings are inspired. It taught me to be in the Here and Now! The *Yoga Anushasan* as taught by Adinath is the mother system from which other *yogachara* systems have branched off. Naga Arjuna, a disciple of Gorakshanath, based his *Prajna Paramita* (knowledge to cross the river of *samsara*) on the ancient Nath and Naga Himalayan schools. Even Gautama, the Buddha, a fully enlightened *avatar*, needed outer practical guidance for his inner spiritual recapitulation. He was a disciple of the ancient Nath Yogis Udraka Ramaputra and Aradyakalam. He followed their way and learned the importance of the *satsang* of the Divine.

One day as I sat in meditation I asked, "Oh Lord! Why does the highest Truth have to hide like a tortoise in its shell? Why has God-realization become so difficult? I am at a loss to understand the difficulty entailed in assessing the lightening path of Yoga."

The inner voice of Babaji replied, "The advanced techniques of Yoga work like the excalibur, a double-edged sword. They not only burn your past evil *karma*, but also evolve your spiritual Consciousness. For this, a personal guidance of a Master is necessary. Such Masters are rare, and this is the reason why lightening evolutionary yogas are still not introduced to the common people. They are too fast and too dangerous to be used even by a practitioner of Yoga when not guided by a Guru. Hence, in order to keep a dsiciple from harms way, no one can be entrusted with this Knowledge before his time, until a true Master takes him under his wing."

Incident at Saswad

I had gone to Saswad with a group of my disciples. In the night a strong urge hit me. So I took the car impulsively to the temple at Saswad in the middle of the night. It was 2:00 am. I was expecting a lot of resistance because I had a premonition that I would get an experience of Gorakshanath. As soon as I thought of this Shiva temple in Saswad, off I went. On arriving at the ancient temple in the forest, a mad dog rushed at me from the nearby thicket. I hit it with the car jack and the dog went reeling into the bushes. It disappeared with a dark light. It then dawned on me that it was an evil spirit who had taken the form of a dog to bite me. Then I climbed up the steep stairs, went inside the temple and meditated into the night. These experiences were like the animation of a special effects film show. Obviously I had shifted into a different astral dimension.

During my meditation in the night, I would get a sensation of something behind me. Somehow, I got this eerie feeling that there was something following me. I was being stretched to an astrally spooky dimension. When the Divine calls you he also gives you the strength to cope with the present situation, if it's a true calling, and this it was. This Being was at the back, where the *Nandi* bull is. Suddenly, he threw a blanket on me while I was meditating. And though he was not much of a shape, he threw himself on me and my breath stopped. It was quite stifling. I wrestled with this formless entity. I broke through, resumed my normal breathing; and continued with my meditation. I carried on deeper and deeper into the night. After I meditated I got this beautiful out of body experience and in my mind's eye I saw this sacred star. I knew I was not alone.

Then all of a sudden I saw this beautiful woman sitting 15 yards away in front of me. Right in front of me to my right, was the *Shiva Linga* of the Chanda Bateshwar temple. I was doing the *Om Nama Shivaya japa* and this woman came in front. She had a salmon pink *sari* and was exceedingly beautiful. It must have been a quarter to three or something. She was very attractive and was trying to entice me, calling me to get up from my *asana* and go and meet her. "No way I'm going to break my *asana*, it may be anyone," I thought. As I was sitting there, she came closer with just a gentle smile. She came even closer, and beckoning me, suddenly she gave me a full smile. Her teeth were like Dracula teeth. Her canine teeth were a little extended line that of a *dakini*. I knew there was something—my innermost core was telling me. I didn't panic. She came closer and closer. She came up to me and twisted her head. She then put her teeth close to my throat. "*Thaaaan!*" There was a noise, a light like a flashbulb exploding, and then a silent explosion. I was quite blinded by the explosion. After that the woman changed into the great Nath Yogi Chanda Vateshwar. He was a disciple of Gorakshanath who lived for more than 1500 years and is still alive today. So, he was the one testing me all the while.

As I went deeper into meditation, I did *pranam* to him. He blessed me, happy for my courage and my strength. There was no test thereafter. A tremendous light, a tremendous power was in the sanctum of the Shiva temple itself. The high point was the scintillating light of the star, the eternal light of truth. I saw it just for a short while. The Nath

Yogi Chand Deva told me that this was Shiva-Goraksha. I had already figured this out intuitively. This Shiva temple had no *Shiva Linga*. The story is that in days long past the great *yogi Chand Deva* meditated and did *tapas* at this temple. Since Lord Shiva did not appear, in his frustration he yanked out the *Shiva Linga*.

After that, I did my *pranam*, my morning *sadhana*, got in my car and drove back to the guesthouse where the rest of my disciples were. There are two or three spiritual experiences I have had in temples. This one was not the very best of them. It was in the night, and quite a powerful one. The good thing about this experience was that it put me to the utmost test. It strengthened me and gave me a boost in my spiritual evolution. The presence of Gorakshanath and Chand Deva was a wonderful happening in my life.

Hamsanet: My Mission and Work

During my preparation and my days of inner learning, I had to be calm with my mind, observe it, and be a witness to its every thought as I gradually transformed it into crystal Consciousness. I could feel the common connection of my spiritual Consciousness with that of humanity's consciousness. To transmute the minds of sincere seekers of yoga into a higher state of consciousness is the purpose of my work. One of the main aspects of my work is helping disciples and truth seekers to enter the unified state of Consciousness, a state of natural enlightenment. This is my mission and my means, "meditated to the furthering of human awareness and dedicated to serving humanity as my larger Self."

I have developed a spiritual network, a unified Consciousness of my own which allows people to realize that at the level of Soul Consciousness, humanity is one. That is why I am here, to tell you about the *Hamsanet*. The *Hamsanet* is the network of light and breath, which the *Satguru* has formed. These are spiritual lights, a spectrum of rainbow light connecting all sincere seekers of truth on earth.

Now, wherever I go, the cord of light will lengthen, even from across the world, from Arizona to Brazil or to India. The centers of the disciples, those who would like to evolve in this manner, are connected to the centers of the Master and therefore my disciples' minds are united to my mind. These connections are mainly at the three main centers of the navel, the heart, and the third eye. The Master connects with the disciple on these three levels because he has to work on them and evolve them, which tens of thousands all over the world have experienced when I transmit the divine energy of *kundalini* by *shaktipat*. A person will feel the *shaktipat* wherever he or she may be, provided his or her mind is open.

Now how is it possible for me to do this; to give my still-mind of unified Consciousness to many people around the world simultaneously? Suppose there are people in Switzerland, America and India, all sitting for meditation at the same time. I, as a total non-entity, which corresponds to humanity's larger Self, will enter the minds of each individual attuned to me the moment the pre-determined time arrives. It is like a hand clap signal from me, and at that precise moment my consciousness will enter all minds and everyone's minds will transform to partake of the unified Consciousness, thereby validating by personal experience that at the level of Consciousness humanity is one.

So the internal stopwatches of these meditators should be synchronized with my spiritual stopwatch. All will sit together at the same time, which makes this work easier. But we want to advance into a system that can be used for earth peace. If there are people in Russia and America, how will they sit with me? So, those who can sit together will sit. We are trying to serve humanity as our larger Self, and if we are to reach humanity, then we must do this stopwatch synchronization. For those in tune with me, they will feel the unified field of Consciousness. It is for Earth-peace through Self-peace that I am holding Unified Consciousness Conferences (U.C.C's) the world over.

Whether I am in my ordinary state of consciousness or in the consciousness of other people or I am really in a different state of consciousness all together, it appears, by what other people say, that I am not in the normal "intellectual" state of consciousness. I am just in awareness. There is not much of "mind" in me. I was born like this. I am unmindful of many things, which other people are mindful of. This is not to say that I don't have a mind. I do have a mind but it lies subservient to my Soul Consciousness (*buddhi*), which is the *connectus conarsus* of the unity in diverse minds.

So, while one mind is in unified Consciousness, all minds tuned to it will be in the unified field of Consciousness (*unmani avastha*), because that is the level at which we're all one. Not at the level of clothes, because one person has a gray outfit, another red maroon, and I have a white one. We are not one at the level of clothes, nor are we onc at the level of the physical body. Everyone is different at the physical level, and our emotions are also different. Then, at what level is humanity one? What is the *connectus conarsus*? What is the common factor of humanity? The answer is simple. At the level of Consciousness, humanity is at-one-ment and peace with itself.

That is the work I do for earth-peace through Self-peace. If we're all in nothing but peace of mind there can be nothing but Earth Peace, not at any contradictory or conflicting level of vibration, but only in the synchronized state of the still-mind can there be a unified consciousness for earth peace and goodwill to all mankind. I say that, "by practice, expand your consciousness to merge with humanity's consciousness and know that your consciousness and humanity's consciousness is one." That's what my services are to humanity. This is highlighted in the Declaration of Human Rights for Earth Peace.

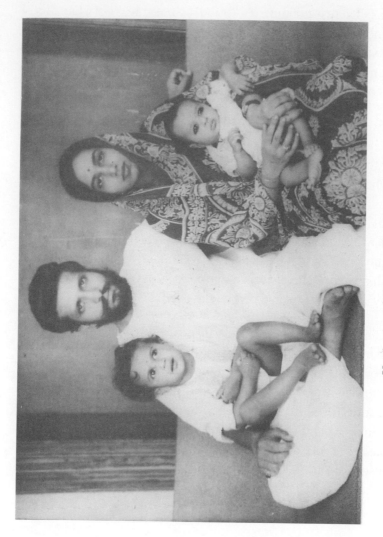

Yogiraj with his family circa 1980
From left: elder son Shivraj, spouse Shivangini and Rudrasen

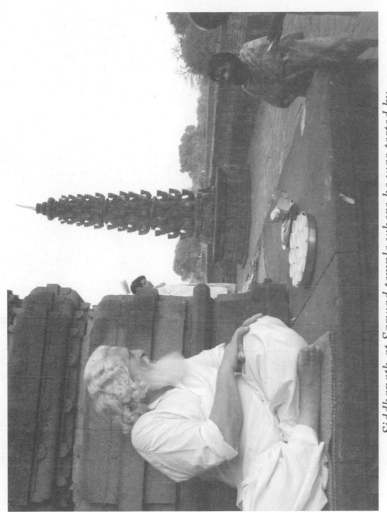

Siddhanath at Saswad temple where he was tested by the great Nath Yogi Chand Deva, a disciple of Babaji

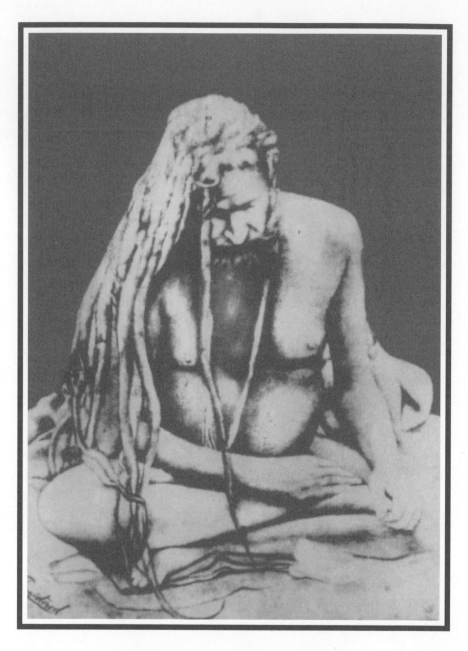

Himalayan Yogi Raja Sundernath
From Siddha to Avadhoot to Avatar

CHAPTER 5

LAND OF THE HAMSAS
LAND OF THE BRAVE

Mystical Revelations from Himalayan Masters

I traveled from the foothills of the Himalayas, starting from the sacred city of Haradwar. This city, called the gate of Shiva, was where the *Kumba Mela* (the world's largest spiritual gathering, with over 30 million participants) was held every twelve years. I then proceeded by public bus transport to Hrishikesh, where the *ashrams* of great spiritual masters like Swami Shivananda, Dayanand Saraswati and Ramakrishna offered rich yogic and spiritual learning. It is said that the great king Vikramaditya, the brother of Bhartarinath, rebuilt and renovated the cities of Haradwar and Hrishikesh to accommodate yogis and *sadhus* mainly to facilitate the great *Kumba Mela*.

Next, I traveled to Rudraprayag, the town at the confluence of the Alakhnanda and Mandakini rivers. Here Lord Shiva himself taught the *Ghandharva*, Devarishi Narada, the art of music and the celestial symphonies. The *Shiva Bhakti Sutras* were given here later called the *Narada Bhakti Sutras*. Then I went to Deva and Vishnu Prayags, and from there to the valley of flowers called Nandan Kanan. It is said that two British travelers stumbled upon this beautiful landscape. They saw it in the flowering season when the whole valley flowered, so they called it "The Valley of Flowers". Yogis cannot help laughing at this because during the autumn season, every valley in the mid-Himalayas becomes a valley of flowers. In these valleys the aroma is so otherworldly that it makes you forget this world and its cares.

Going further up into the Garwal Mountains, I came to the foothills of the Badri-Kedar range of the Himalayas. Here the evergreen forest was lush and rivulets of melted ice from the mountains were nectar fresh. Walking on beaten paths leading up to higher regions was like walking towards heaven. With the smell of pine-cones and wild berries, a past life nostalgia arose within me. It wafted me to yogic memories of a land far away yet so near to me. It was the land of the *Hamsas*, the Swans who took flight in *samadhi* to reach their beloved Lord. Such yogis, the *Hamsa Yogis* exist even today in the Himalayan ranges and it is to their abode in the rarer regions that I made my pilgrimage.

They are ever engaged in spiritual practices and meditations, these yogis called *Hamsas*. The *Hamsa* (Soul Swan) is represented as the inhaled and exhaled breath of one's self. The "*Ham*" syllable is meditated upon as our breath is exhaled, and the "*Sah*" is meditated upon as our breath is inhaled. This is a *Hamsa Sadhana* (spiritual practice), laid down in the *yogic* book of the *Gheranda Samhita*. The *Vigyan Bhairava* text says the opposite—inhaled breath is "*Ham*" and exhaled is "*Sah*," but Gorakshanath put an end to the confusion saying that the mental chanting of *Ham-Sah* could be done either way. He emphasized meditating on the still gap between the "*Ham*" and the "*Sah*". As the gap lengthens, our mind stills into consciousness and the yogi achieves *kevali kumbak* to enter *samadhi* of the Here Now!

The *Hamsas* have given up *samsara* (all worldly ways or pleasures) to seek God. Making the search for God, their life's only goal, they practice the *Hamsa* breath (*pranayama*) and meditation night & day. These lofty beings bless and evolve all humanity by their spiritual vibrations. Their miniature counterparts and representatives are the *yogacharya* and *hamsacharya* schools of teachers who help in the evolution of human consciousness by teaching *Hamsa Yoga*, *Kriya Yoga*, *Bhakti Yoga* and *Raja Yoga*.

Now I had already traveled quite a distance along the path to Badrinath, at times by public transport, and at times by hitch hiking. As it was not in my nature to travel much, I tarried for two days at all of these small pilgrimage confluences. My last stop was Hanuman Chatti and then I arrived at the great playground of Shiva, called Badrinath. "What's life about anyway?" I mused. Suddenly I felt myself a dream within a dream universe.

The universe but a pale phantom of a deeper order,
Oh Lord only thou dost know thine own awesome
reality!

There is a legend that Vishnu loved Badrinath and wished to dwell there. Shiva did not take Vishnu's wish seriously and was lost in *samadhi* for the salvation of existence. So Vishnu took the form of an infant crying in the snowy mountains. Parvati, the consort of Shiva, saw the child and her heart melted. She nurtured Vishnu with love until he grew up. Then both Shiva and Parvati, out of love for their adopted child, gave him the pilgrimage place of Badrinath. Here Vishnu, in the form of the sage Narayana, is established in *yoga-samadhi* for the salvation of *Bharat Varsha* (India) and humanity.

This legend, of course, has deeper cosmic and philosophical implications, such as the evolution of both Nara and Narayana. There is also the series of *avataric* incarnations of Narayana to assist in the spiritual evolution of humanity.

The first day at Badrinath I visited the temple, paid my respects to Sanatana Rishi Narayan, then went to pay my respects to the photo of the monumental *Siddha* Sundernath, as I was honored to belong to and be blessed by his *parampara* and lineage of Masters of the Babaji Gorakshanath tradition. The legendary *yogi* Sundernath meditated in a cave near the temple of Badrinath. I had the good fortune to visit the cave hallowed by this great *Siddha*. Before I entered the cave, I saw in front of it a Margosa tree. It was bent in the same meditation posture as the yogi. This tree usually has bitter leaves, but as I broke the leaves off the tree and put them in my mouth, to my surprise they tasted sweet. This brought to mind that a similar such tree with sweet leaves is near the *samadhi of* Shirdi Baba, in the town of Shirdi in Maharastra. Shirdinath is now with the celestial group of Shiva-Goraksha-Babaji.

As I entered the cave I had to bend low. In front of me to the right was an earthen oven to cook food. To my extreme left was a raised rock platform, and to the interior left was another meditation *samadhi* place. With reverence I sat down and the powerful currents of the lofty Sundernath engulfed me. Within moments I was gone from myself. I was not able to have the much desired vision of this great yogi. But I did receive his blessings in the form of dazzling light, which pushed my consciousness to higher dimensions. I felt renewed and deeply privileged at having been able to meditate in the hallowed cave of the Divine Master.

From Badrinath, I set out on my sojourn and search for the *Hamsas* and the land of the *Hamsas*. "Where is this place?" I wondered. Is it true or just stories told by our parents? How could these yogis survive in such cold snowy regions? All these questions rushed to my mind as I lay asleep before my morning journey to Vasundhara waterfalls, Chakratirth and Satopant glacier. I got up early and braced myself for the trek, heading for the little Indo-Tibetan village of Mana. On reaching it, I found the Indian army had camped in the village as the China border was near. From Mana I headed to Bhimpool, a bridge where I had a glorious sight of the river Saraswati rushing out of the snowy mountains as white as milk, with tremendous force. I inhaled the power of wisdom from the Saraswati, bowed and moved on towards the falls.

I was now at 11,000 feet or so and the air had naturally become rarer. At last I beheld the Vasundhara falls with bated breath. The beautiful river Alaknanda melted from the Satopant glacier and flowed over the mountain top as a waterfall.

It was along these tracks that I came upon the wonderful *Hamsa Yogis*. One yogi, Balak Bairagi, told me that all along the Badri-Kedar tracks, right up to Gangotri and Jamnotri, yogis like himself meditated during summer. It was at an altitude of eight to twelve thousand feet that they lived and meditated. When winter came, most of them descended to lower altitudes of five to seven thousand feet, but some still remained at the higher altitudes during winter. Government officials, like collectors, have reported having seen them in winter, and some yogis have been known to go up to those heights to supply food. They practice the *Hamsa* meditation as I explained before. The Bairagi yogi told me that they practiced the *kumbaka* (retention of breath) *pranayama* with the *Hamsa* breath. They alternated it with the *Hamsa* of the watchful breath. Becoming proficient in the science *of kundalini pranayama,* and balancing the breath, they entered *samadhi*.

Samadhi is a supra-consciousness state of ecstasy. The restless mind, the yogis say, contains all sorrow and unfulfilled desires. They transform the desire-filled mind to supra-consciousness and enter into supreme consciousness, a state of blissful God communion. I was deeply moved and wonder-struck by the simplicity of their lifestyle and purpose of life. As I left to go, the Balak Bairagi yogi offered me some roots of shrubs, which I ate. Surprisingly, I felt rejuvenated and full of energy a few minutes after I had eaten them. Then he told me to go and visit a place of caves called the Chakra Tirtha, so I set out, my eyes filled with wonder and my heart full of love for these Himalayan *Hamsas*. When I reached Chakra Tirtha, there were caves and water-flows, and I came to a cave covered by a flowing waterfall. The waterfall formed the curtain of the cave. Behind the waterfall of the cave lived a yogi. Not knowing his true name, people called him *Khadeswar Nath Baba* or just Baba. This means "the standing Lord Father."

So I sat outside the cave, waiting for him to come. I remembered again my own past life as a yogi meditating in these regions. In this life I did the same, but it was not as continuous as before. My work was to teach people in daily life and in the lower altitude cities.

"Not so good for me," I thought. An hour passed and nothing happened. I heard the cracking and crashing sound of huge ice slabs as they fell into the rivers and streams in the vicinity. At this altitude there were no trees, only shrubs and further on, no vegetation at all. It was near the snowline of the Himalayas. Yogis follow the snowline during all seasons. This keeps them at constantly cool temperature, which assists them to practice Yoga and also to arrest the aging process of their body cells.

As I reveled in my thoughts, I felt a great calm energy surrounding me. I opened my eyes and beheld the yogi. He came out from behind the waterfall. He was standing with one arm raised above his head. "My God!" I exclaimed to myself, "is this the true form of the great yogi whose pictures I had often seen as a child?" They were doing *tapasya,* which literally signifies heat or fire, and implies the ordeal of spiritual transformation where the *tapasvi* or yogi stews in his own juices to transform himself. *Tapa* means to deliberately create dissatisfaction with life, for lacking God. "No God, no life," says the *tapasvi*, so he kicks up a row with the elements, showing his yearning and burning for God. Oh what a way to go! The Naths and Aghoris are *tapasvis* too!

The practice of austerities is done for the sake of God. These pains were undertaken in order to commune with God. "Oh, the passion of it all!" I thought. I wondered if there is any other place on earth where people laid their lives on the line for the love of God. It is difficult to feel the intensity of the passion they must generate in their quest for the Absolute! And this is not one person, mind you. There are many such sons of God making their way back home with a lightning rapidity and intense God-yearning. This passion for God in which India specializes, is not of one generation, but of generation after generation of people, who renounce their worldly vocations and set out in search for God. The common lot of the people in India is like that of any other people, anywhere in the world. They are very family oriented, with strong family ties. The richer class loves the good things of life. Family quarrels and love affairs are abundant, but they do not reflect nor represent the class of yogis and ascetics. Though these yogis rise from among our common people, they are yet a breed apart. Even if such people are few and far between, their types have never died. As long as such noble souls strive for the Divine, that's how long there will be hope for our people on this planet.

As I got nearer to this yogi, Khadeshwar Baba, a deep profundity of peace surrounded him. My mind melted into awareness and I forcefully kept thinking of questions to ask him.

"What do you do all day?" I asked.

"Be with God," was the simple reply.

"Why do you keep your hand above your head?"

"It is God's will I have surrendered to."

"And does your body take any stance he wants you to take?" Again he smiled and said, "Yes!" I then asked if initially he made the effort by *tapa* to keep his hand up.

"Yes," he replied, "but I now flow."

"You mean now you have surrendered yourself to God?" He smiled and gave no reply.

I let half an hour pass before I gingerly put my question to him. "Do you go to the Shiva temple of Kedar Nath?"

"When he summons me I go," was his response.

Now the standing yogi's peace vibrations had become overwhelmingly peaceful. I found myself slipping into meditation. A great comfort of mind enveloped me and I was gone. How long I meditated on the rocks before the cave, I have no idea. When I opened my eyes I was alone, and the yogi had gone into his cave. I thought to myself that this great *tapasvin* did not sit down, but must be directly lying down to sleep. Little did I realize that such beings have totally sacrificed themselves at the altar of God's love and did not sleep but went into *samadhi*. But with the thought—who knows and who can tell—I set out on my Himalayan trek in the land of the *Hamsas*.

It is said that when Sundernath undertook his *tapas* in a cave near Badrinath temple, the Badrinath vibrated with his spiritual intensity.

One day some miscreants (they were just boys we were told) went into the cave and found Raja Sundernath in *samadhi*. To test his yogic state of trance they placed a burning charcoal on his thigh. The king of yogis didn't budge for he was totally out of his body in *samadhi*, so the burning coal went deep into his thigh. On descending from his heightened state of awareness, the yogi saw his thigh all burnt. With compassion, he blessed the boys, for they had created a context whereby Yogi Sundernath knew that he could never be shaken or diverted from his practice and communion with God. It is said that this great master traveled into the solitudes of the higher regions of the Himalayas, to the legendary city of Alkapuri. This spiritual center near the Indo-China border is where he is lost in communion with God.

The air was getting rarer as I climbed higher. I had heard of the city of Alkapuri and dared to think of visiting that place where the lofty *Siddhas* reside. As I trudged through the snowy terrain, my mind got very volatile due to the rarity of oxygen. At times my thought process dissolved and I found myself in rarer states of mind. I was then able to perceive life and beings in other worldly dimensions. I continued with my meditations, to keep myself balanced. So my journey towards the city of Alkapuri and my meditations both went on with equal enthusiasm. I meditated on Yogi Sundernath, that he would meet me during my journey. But traveling in the snowy terrain I was soon exhausted and lay down to twilight sleep in a nearby shelter. My sleep was a bit insufficient. I had a vision of a yogi with long dreadlocks who told me with a sign of his index finger that I should not continue towards Alkapuri, but he gave me no reasons. So when I awoke, my feet turned towards the sacred pilgrimage of Shiva at Kedar Nath instead. From there I was planning to go to the origin of the Ganges river (called Gangotri) and then to the source of the Yamuna river, Yamnotri—both sacred places to the *Hamsas*.

It was like awakening into new life as I made my way towards the higher regions of Mount Kedar. I had enough rations with me but I couldn't eat much. I walked on for a day, all the while breathing "Shiva" with every breath, and reached Kedar Nath. As I crossed a ravine, I saw some glorious yogis of unearthly appearance who greeted me with, "*Ram! Ram!*" I said the same.

Seeing these lofty *yogis* I remembered the likes of Rishi Narayana, Shiva-Goraksha-Babaji, Vishwamitra and Dhruva. My heart sank at the sight of the dizzying heights achieved by these greats yogis present before me, and those great yogis gone before us in robes of light. "Could we all achieve these states of God-Realization?" I asked myself. I had by now almost become a non-entity in their presence.

I was tired and disheveled-looking like them. And why not, was I not a yogi too? I asked them who they were and they said they were *Hamsas* and expounded the *Raja Yoga* and *Hamsa Sadhana* of Babaji Goraknath. As they said this, they looked at one of the silent figures seated in the background, who appeared very ethereal to my sight.

I humbly requested them to bless me and to teach me the Yoga of Babaji. The youngest and most junior of these lofty yogis taught me a form of *Kundalini Kriya Yoga* and *Raja Yoga*. Even while I was learning, by their grace, my mind entered supra-conscious states of ecstasy. I was seeing those *yogis* being transformed into Babaji and Sundernath. I couldn't figure out if this was true or whether I was hallucinating, since I was still not acclimatized to this altitude and my mind would sort of expand out into dimensions beyond my comprehension. These rarer states of mind offered no support for my rationality, of which I had very little in any case.

I had been traveling a day from Vasundhara Falls and was now exhausted. The yogis gave me some roots and herbs to eat which revived me for my journey. They blessed me and said the meditation on Mahadeva (Shiva) would evolve me fast.

As I walked, I remembered that Sundernath himself was a member of the *Satnath* section of *Goraknathis*. The Gorakshanath

Babaji yogic tree has twelve branches, *Satnath* being one of them. They say the lineage descended from Adinath (*Shiva* himself), who gave it to Parvati-Nath (his consort), who gave it to her two sons Kanthadnath and Kartikeya. This divine science of Yoga was further passed onto Vishnu who initiated the spirit of our sun called Vaivashvat, and from there it descended to the kings of the solar dynasty who guarded and preserved this science from age to age. From Vaivashvat Surya, Vaivashvat Manu got the initiation and then gave the science of the evolution of consciousness to Ikshavaku. It was then passed on to Raghu, then Dilip and later to Harischandra, and then to Rama, 37th in descent from Ikshavaku.

Shiva-Goraksha-Babaji—The Eternal Now—is a direct manifestation of Adinath Shiva, himself and it is he who has enlightened the modern age with this soul liberating science. It is to this grand lineage or *parampara* that I belong and am privileged to teach the science of Kriya Yoga as a "Servant of Humanity". All the Yogas, like *Raja Yoga, Kriya Yoga, Bhakti Yoga, Jnana Yoga, Karma Yoga, Hatha Yoga, Laya Yoga, Tantra Yoga* and *Hamsa Yoga* come from the same source, for the blessings and salvation of all humankind. This is a non-denominational, non-sectarian way of life which compliments all faiths and religions and contradicts none.

As I was in an expanded state of awareness, the cold and discomfort of these regions did not bother me. I had no idea how I stayed or how long I stayed with these yogis. All I knew was that they protected and taught me what I was destined to learn. I noticed that the person who had transformed into Babaji never taught anything but was always "The Silent Watcher", immovable, immaculate and eternal-looking. Was he even a being or just a figment of my imagination? No sooner had I thought this, then the voiceless voice of the Babaji figure echoed in my soul, "The whole universe is a figment of God's imagination. To get to reality transcend name and form!" The other Nath Yogi, Sundernath, waved his hand over my head and I got the realization of a unified field of Consciousness, that my Consciousness and that of humanity's is One. In yogic parlance this is known as the state of *asmita samadhi*. This is the generic pool of all individualized consciousness of humanity.

Then a very strange thing happened which, for reasons unknown to me, I have kept secret until now. As the third great *yogi* approached me, he was transformed into Priya Nath, who is Gyanavatar Yukteswar (meaning the incarnation of wisdom). "Oh," I thought, "you were on *Hiranyaloka* teaching Yoga to *Paramahamsas* and *Siddhas*!" I was surprised to see his divine presence here in the land of the *Hamsas*, but he had come to give me the state of ecstasy experienced in *Hiranyaloka*. With a glance he let me to know that although the heavenly spheres were real places, they could also be experienced in supra-conscious states of *samadhi*.

Next he came in a glorious form and engulfed me in his aura. My conscious ecstasy of being one with the Consciousness of humanity was transformed into a No-Thing-Ness. My former state of *asmita samadhi* took subtler wings into a flight I am incapable of describing. But however imperfectly, I shall try:

Samadhi

O Thou phantom of creation's song
Why did you keep me tied so long?

This nature's Eve, she can't deceive
The people pure and strong

For they in God's own light perceive
The truth where they belong.

I stop this breath, my stillness enters
Into the velvety darkness of death.

I grow in consciousness sublime
Engulfing countries, continents and time.

I further grow in omniscient glow
To unite with maya's karmic flow.

The subtle laws of cause and effect
Within myself I do detect.

Beyond the gates of death! I glide – untied;
Into regions sublime – surpassing causation,
Space and time.

Here Eternal Bliss is King by name of Sat Chit Anand
Whose Life Divine is Loving Brahmanand.

I fill immensity of space – I am the Self Supreme
Looking down I do perceive creation as a dream.

I then blend in the everlasting expanse of Lightless Light
Beyond the Cosmic Hum of all resounding ...
Ommmmmm

My consciousness expanded and became aware of the vaster realms of knowingness. This is what is called the yogic state of *asamprajnata samadhi*. In Vedantic terms, it is known as *nirvikalpa samadhi*. Our consciousness slumbers in matter, and as it ascends to mind, it awakens. When it transcends mind to dwell in Soul consciousness, it is enlightened.

You see that consciousness is the substratum of the universe, without which nothing can exist nor not exist. This makes us question whether consciousness is an integral part of God playing the eternal witness, as well as the eternal catalyst, changing the whole universe and its material manifestations, transforming and evolving all matter and mind and yet remaining the same. Yes, this is true, so when consciousness withdraws itself from the grosser sheaths of matter, through subtler sheaths of mind, it evolves both of them and itself becomes more and more expressive of its omnipresent and omniscient Self until it merges into the ultimate God-essence—its own True Self, an *avasta* of supreme conscious ecstasy.

After that, I went to Tunganath and passed my days assimilating my experiences and my realizations. Tunganath is a name of Lord Shiva meaning, "Lord of Strong Arms." This temple is situated at an altitude of about 12,000 ft and is one of the highest in those regions. From there I climbed down to the valley of Duggal-bitha at 8,500 ft, and passed a few days meditating in the quiet mountains.

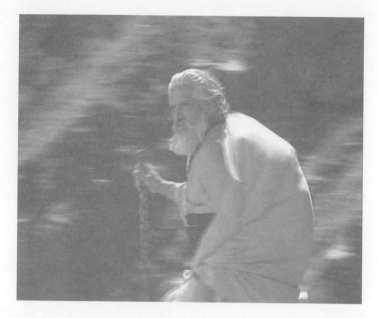

Yogiraj revisiting the Himalayas for a documentary film

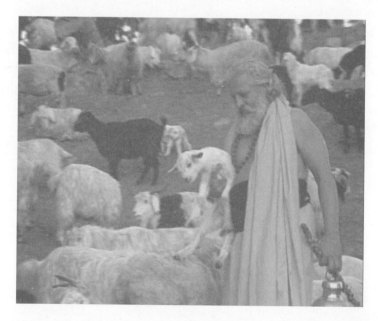

Yogiraj as a Servant of Humanity - shepard for lost lambs

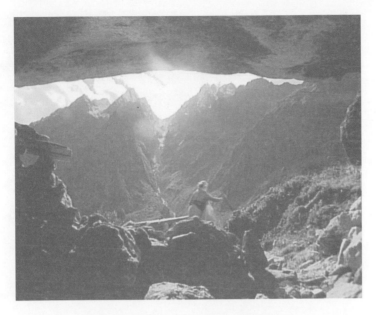

*Walking to Vasundhara Falls in
the Himalayan land of the Hamsas*

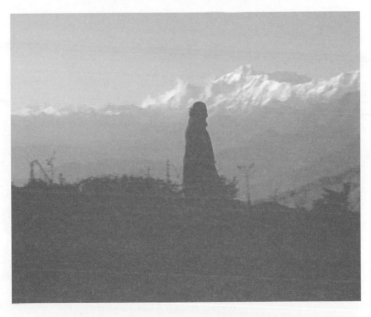

Yogiraj traversing the Himalayan ranges

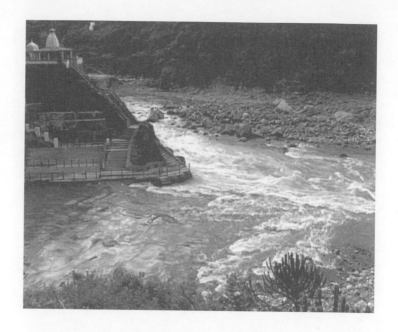

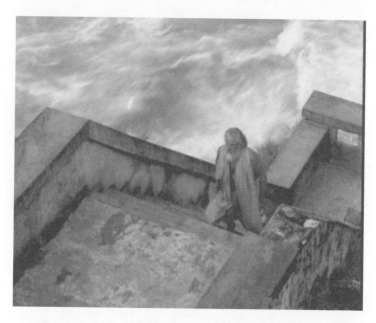

Yogiraj at Rudraprayag
The sacred confluence of the Alakhnanda and Mandakini rivers

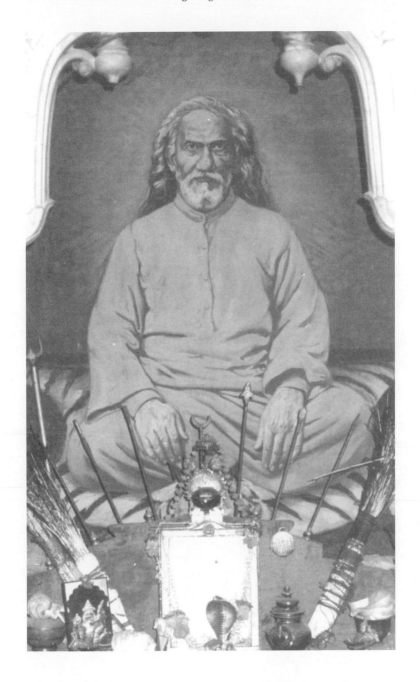

Gyana Avatar Shri Yukteswar, an incarnation of Wisdom.

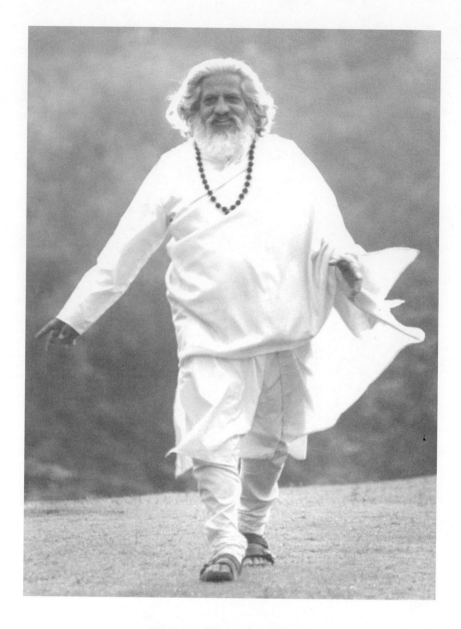

*Yogiraj: Sanatana Hamsa
conducting a New Life Awakening Camp*

CHAPTER 6

MEETING WITH DIVINE BEINGS AND YOGIS OF THE HIMALAYAS

All throughout my school and college days I came into personal and visionary contact with great Himalayan sages and *yogis*. One of the most remarkable features of these *anubhutis*, that surprised me, is that they occurred at times in the most commonplace circumstances and places, where I least expected to have them. The vision would burst upon my sight carrying me into dimensions that were para-normal, but real all the same. What was most intriguing to me was that when I was getting an experience, I was giving an experience to others simultaneously.

I shall now go on to relate some of my meetings and experiences, to inspire people to believe that Divine Beings exist, and to practice the art of evolution. I myself am deeply convinced that if any student of Yoga practices with earnest regularity, he shall not only attract the blessings of the Masters, but also progress towards Self-realization. Experiences are benchmarks to spur the individual soul in its evolutionary path. All those who meditate with single-minded purpose shall be blessed by their guiding Masters. They will get inspirational experiences according to their evolutionary needs.

The eight *siddhis** also manifest according to the spiritual evolution of the particular soul. These super normal powers distract a soul from his main path to Self-realization and must not be indulged in by the soul. But an adept, who is realized, may use the *siddhis* for the welfare of humanity and especially for the spiritual progress of his disciples.

The Rudraprayag Experience

Once again, I traveled on to the Himalayas to search for the Beloved of my heart. Call him the "Nameless One," call him "the Lightening Standing Still," the "Lord of Irradiant Splendor"—Shiva Goraksha. As I climbed into the uncharted regions, I had no doubt that my feet were set upon the right path, and whether I would achieve or not achieve was not an issue with me. I would still go to the spot where I wanted to go and be absorbed in the *Paramatma* essence. Walking and meditating, I went up to this confluence of the Alakhananda and Mandakini rivers called Rudraprayag. It was a full moon night. I had heard stories of sages and great masters, the great Divine Beings who came and bathed at the confluences. I had heard stories from the Super-conscious spheres of my mind, from yogis, from *sadhus* and sages about the wonders of the places in the Himalayas. Places like Panch Kashi, Panch Kedar and Panch Prayag are sacred to the pilgrims and yogis.

So I went and started settling down at Rudraprayag. There I got deeper into my meditation and *sadhana*. Then came the night of the full moon and, as I observed the gurgling of the Alakhananda mixing with the soft Mandakini river, my mind melted into the water. I waited and waited, and then I had the experience of my life.

---

*The *siddhis* are the powers of the Yogi's soul as he progresses in his spiritual and evolutionary practice. The freer he is from material desires the more he expresses the super natural powers. According to the *Yoga Bhasya*, there are 8 principal *siddhis*. They are 1) *Animan* (to become as small or smaller than an atom, 2) *Lahiman* (Lighter than air Levitation), 3) *Mahiman* (Magnification to infinitely larger size, 4) *Prapte* (to get whatever wanted), 5) *Prakamya* (Irresistible will), 6) *Vashitva* (Mastery over anyone), 7) *Ishitritva* (Lordship over the universe), 8) *Kama Avasayitva* (fulfillment of desires). The fickle minded should not dwell upon the *mahasiddhis*. Only a *Siddha* may use them for the benefit of progressing other souls along the spiritual path.

As I meditated, my consciousness expanded, and suddenly the river was flowing right through my stomach, up my spine, and merging into the third eye. My awareness grew into the night as I waited in an indescribable state. I waited in a state of awareness, which I was not able to decipher or know. Everything around me became oblivious and I entered a steady gaze called *shambhave*. But in my case, I was looking from within - without. The outer became the inner and inner became the outer, such that my Self turned inside out. I again and again tell you that it's very difficult for me to explain spiritual experiences in material and physical words. But in my broken way, and inadequate language, I have to do it.

So my innermost core became my outermost being and my outermost portion became the innermost being. Nature became within me. The trees, the hills, the snow, were all inside me and I was turned inside out. Now in this state, as I waited, there was a glow of light, a lilac light, very soft yet very iridescent in its splendor. I saw it coming along. This light came closer and closer. It was like a whirl, a lilac color, a blue, and an indigo color. I do not know what precise color it was. It was a color for which we have no name on this earthly plane. In the center it became whiter and whiter and lighter and lighter. That formation was Infinity—was Nothingness, the indescribable seed of Nothingness from which the Infinite creation had sprung.

It made me feel as though I had met my innermost being. That light was so revolving, like an aurora borealis, with all the splendor of the Northern Lights and more. It was radiating and washing the whole countryside. It washed and flooded the whole place, even more than the river, and flooded my body. Like a drunken madman was my state. This is the closest description. So when you are in that state, all these little rough edges and discomforts vanish. You are just floating; you are going with the universal flow of livingness.

It was as though this mysterious Being that came, the Absolute, Shiva-Goraksha-Babaji, was giving this experience to himself. It means he had illumined my core being by his grace, taken me to an egoless state where I felt that I myself and that light were the same. It was the Self giving the *self* an experience. And it was He, not me. Sometimes you get an experience that the light is you and the body is you, giving an experience to yourself. But it was he giving an experience to Himself as me.

I was reveling in a state of my own. I did not lose my identity, but I was more than my own. I was his Consciousness and identity, twinkling in the stars, rushing in the river of the Alakhananda, flowing gently and softly in the feminine nature of the Mandakini. It was like a union of the Shiva and Shakti. As the light actualized into a "Non-being Essentiality," the essence of a nothing, whose majesty ignited all creation; *before whose coming the whole of nature and creation stood in awe with folded hands and bowed head.*

A yogi, they say, is very powerful, forceful, and that makes it appear that he is very egotistic, but he is not. It is just the way he moves, the way he is. He is not proud, but humble. Let there come a situation where he can be humble and bow his head, and it will automatically bow. So when this happened, his Divinity and gravity automatically bowed my head. I was in a headless state. I surrendered. Then there was a blinding flash. It was a lightless flash deep in its splendor. It was the mother of all light. It was the fathomless deep. So, this "Lightless Light," which lights that light, which lights the light of all our Souls, was this indescribable Light; a great nothingness of such Truth that it was immaterial.

No matter how many descriptive words we use, we will always fall into the pit of ignorance. Get the best linguist, get the best sophist, and we will still be hopelessly tongue-tied. We will fail. The silence prevailed, and when this "Lightless Light" came, a past life experience flowed into this life experience. When I go into certain stages, my *avastas* blend into one another. My past life comes rushing in to merge with this life and it is then difficult to distinguish whether I was Rana

Rudrasen Singh Rawal of a past life or Siddhanath of this life. This happens sometimes.

It must have been a state of *nirvikalpa samadhi*. Even though the *nirvikalpa samadhi* was given to me by a grace, the grace is not something that you get idly. The Divine Masters or the *avatars* do not simply come, bestow grace, and give you *samadhi*. They give it to you because you loved and practiced yoga in your past life. It is a well-deserved spiritual harvest that you reap. Put your shoulder to the wheel of *sadhana*, practice and love. I believe that to each one is meted out his exact and proper due. Otherwise everyone would say, "In any case, Shiva is going to give me *samadhi*, so what are these yogis doing in the Himalayas meditating? Let us have wine, women, laughter, sermons and soda water the day after!" Everybody would do it. Why strive? Why make the necessary sacrifice? So it is a wrong mindset and philosophy to be lazy. You have to be assiduous and practice. Be pure, go in the direction of your spiritual practice of *Shiva-Shakti*, do Babaji's *Kriya Yoga* and the fruit will be yours in this life and the next.

So when this blinding light flashed, I blanked out. I am unable to describe what had happened. When I came to, I was lying on the ground with the stars in the sky. I saw that the flash had materialized as a body—the body was Divine Lightless Light, which he had taken for human understanding, for limited minds and intellect of human beings. The Nameless One, the Non-Being! According to my past *samskaras*, he was Gorakshanath. Whatever your limited mind makes of the divine, that it shall be for you. It was a wondrous state. I just let things happen. There was nothing on my part that I could do. He came, climbed up to a certain place where there was a hut-like thing, and he said, "Come and sit down." What they (the Divine Beings) say happens; it is the truth. The bell rang at Shiva's temple. Whatever Babaji says shall come to pass; anything uttered from Soul-Consciousness, from Divine Consciousness, and he *is* Divine Consciousness, the Infinite personified. If he said, "Let there be light," in the darkest night the sun would have to come up and obey. But these Beings do not break the laws, which they have created themselves. If they were led by moods and whims there would be chaos in the cosmos.

He came very simply and sat down, and I was sitting before him. When I gazed into him, I didn't know what happened. What was the depth, what was the infinity? I had no idea, not a clue. It was like peering into *Amba*, "the great deep." He said, "Take this onion and take this seed." I am using words but sometimes my mind blanks out. I was not paying attention to what he was saying. I was more engrossed in drinking his eyes, in drinking him in. I was quenching my thirst of the ages. I said words do not matter, because in any case, he had a double back-up system, just like when you record a person you have a dictaphone and you have a video as well. If one doesn't work, you have the other.

He was telling me in words and putting encapsulated light photons into my memory bank while he was talking. He said, "You know the seed. Take this seed of a vast tree and break it". I did so and found in its innermost core a hollow-space. Some onions happened to be lying there. He took an onion. "Peel It," said he. So I went on peeling it. "Peel it more." And I peeled it more. I was enjoying it, you know. I wondered, "That's some task he's given me. I'm not Secretary General of the U.N. I'm not a big officer in a company with big responsibilities…I'm not anybody. Here I am, peeling onions." I didn't even have time—because the import of the thing was such that I forgot who I was sitting in front of, what his majesty, what his power was, because if I'd known this I would have dissolved. Had this Being, this Presence expressed what he truly was, I would have evaporated in sheer Truth. It's like lightning striking you. What are you? Where are you? You would just have gone. Nothing remains.

He accommodated himself to my limited understanding, although he had expanded it sufficiently into states of *samadhi*. He had an important lesson to teach and I went on peeling the onion. It was like peeling off the delusive layers of my mind. Then he said, "Peel the last." I peeled the innermost core and there was space. He asked, "What's in there?" So I said, "Nothing." Then he said, "My son, the Truth of all truths is this: that from the Nothing is the Everything created." His words gave me the realization that when the universe and its coats of illusion (that is *maya*) are peeled off, you get pure Consciousness, which to the material world is nothing. It is totally immaterial. And from that nothing does the whole of Creation arise. He laughed! I do not know what happened after that for when he laughed I passed out and was not aware of myself. Later, when I regained normal consciousness, I realized with gratitude the knowledge given to me. So much river had run by, so many stars in the sky. The holy men had lit their night fires on the mountains.

It was after this expansion that I was able to give *unmani*, the experience of my unified consciousness to all sincere and receptive seekers of Truth! Here the mind heightens and expands into its own state of awareness. Everything gets altered. Time and space dissolve. These things happen out of mind. We should make a language that is simple and the message will be clear. My bestowing of unified Soul-consciousness of thoughtless awareness is best understood by experiencing it.

I was saying that when the light came, the aurora borealis, and then Babaji appeared. He was experiencing himself because there was none of me left. But if that was the case, then how am I recalling this to you? So he had heightened my awareness to a little of his consciousness, which I now share universally. Then it was I experiencing myself as part of him. The yogis experience this beautiful thing called "stargate". We go into something Infinite. When we pass through "stargate," we go to another dimension, where time and cognition are not. It is sheer essence, a flavor, an aroma. It's a vast expanse going to deep space and beyond, through the "stargate" into the essence of non-being. And then such a voltage! It is a tremendous light that actually transforms.

95

Meeting with Anandamayi Ma

True to her name she was the joy permeated mother. Oblivious to the thousands of devotees who thronged to her, she was ever engrossed in the Lord. She was visiting Pune, my hometown in India, in the year 1970. The monsoons had set in, I remember, and the word was in the air that the Mother was in town.

It was on a Sunday that I was meditating in my underground cellar. I was not motivated to see her because of the rush of devotees who crowded her ashram. As my meditation deepened, there emerged from my inward eye the smiling face of Ma. She was beckoning me to come and see her. I perceived in my meditation a long line of devotees with me in the line. As I approached closer to her she leaned aside, looked at me and smiled. She then took a white garland of fragrant flowers and threw it at me. They hit my chest and came into my hands and she said, "Come!" I mentally said, "okay, it's just a mental image," but as I opened my eyes to my delight her face still persisted smiling, alive and very real.

So after my meditation I set out to meet the Divine Mother and waited my turn in a queue for her *darshan* (blessings with her sight). As I approached her, she leaned aside, smiled, took the white garland of flowers and threw it at me. The flowers hit my chest and came into my hands. My meditation had become a reality. Soon in her presence she touched my head and said, "God looks to them that look at him," and her chant of *Hari Bol* continued. She then stopped and after a while went into a glorious state of *nirvikalpa samadhi*. The whole ambience and audience were transported with her to another world.

I spent entire days at Ma's ashram in great peace, often finding a spot to meditate, often not. So the day passed on. It was evening and Ma was sitting outside her room on a divan. All the people and devotees were sitting around her as she became quiet and went into *khayal* (a state of deep introspection). We all felt the breeze bringing a sultry message of rain. The clouds arrived large and dark portending a heavy shower as everybody became restless for the Mother, that she should not get soaked in the rain. But she was as serene and calm as ever, not moving at all. The forked lightning lit up the clouded sky, as the clouds threateningly rumbled to rain down upon us. Then suddenly a downpour of rain began. Ma transfixed the skies for a while, and sat silent, lost in her own *avasta* (state of consciousness). Lo and Behold! Was I seeing what I was seeing? The rain showered all around us but not a drop of rain in the *ashram* area. Now, to my mind, this was a miracle, a *siddhi* she performed. But to her it was merely a spontaneous happening with no conscious effort on her part. This taught me the great lesson of life, "The more you trust in God, the more trustable He becomes."

A few days later by her grace I was able to meet her. She told me, "Don't be impressed by such miracles but, by the lessons they teach. In the future, as you travel the world to teach, you too will be able to command the elements, to inspire the confidence of God in people." With this she got up and went into her room. The words of such an *avatar* are never empty. A few years later a similar stopping of the rain by me occurred at the ashram of Dhundi Baba at Ram Dara near Pune. Arvind Rane and Baba Sathe were witness to this event. My "I" however had no hand or ego in the happening. The power of the elements was within me, and to remove their doubts, the rain stopped on the hillock where we were, while all round the hillock it rained.

The next incident was when I was on Long Island teaching a group of lesbians. The Divine created a thunderstorm through me to cure the "Doubting Thomas'" of their skepticism in yogis and all healers of humanity. That incident removed their blocks and healed many of them.

I often wondered why these incidents took place through me when I least expected them to. An uncanny force welled up within and with great spontaneity I was able to do what was to be done. It was to inspire the confidence of the God-Essence in them and speed them on their path of evolution. It is indeed very awkward for me to pen down such supernatural events as they appear to smack of a certain pride or boast. But at the command of the Master I am told to write, and so I write. As one grows upon the spiritual path, supernatural events become natural, and *siddhis* (as they are called) may be used for the service of humanity, to inculcate faith in them and their evolution. They may be brought into play at the behest of the Master for reasons best known to him. But they must never be used for self-aggrandisement as they delude the Soul from its journey to God.

Getting back to Anandamayi Ma—she is the greatest of women of grace and glory. I reflect here also on the spiritual stature of my own mother, who in her naïve innocence created a permanent place in many hearts. Such was her purity that once when she came out of our family temple with the *aarti*, through the flaming lamps, I saw in her the actual blaze and form of the Goddess Ambika. This was no hallucination. It was 10 o'clock in the morning. Her crystal heart was so newborn that whatever she said came to pass. The same dazzling form of the Goddess Ambika I saw in Anandamayi Ma. I was shocked at the similarity of my experience because I considered my mother to be just an ordinary good householder lady. But I was proven wrong—strange are the ways of the Lord, beyond mortal comprehension. Anandamayi Ma, my ceaseless salutations to thee. My dear mother (Snehalata was her name), ceaseless salutations to Thee. My mother's experience is a very personal one, so why did I write it? I don't know, just a happening of my pen I suppose.

Experience with The Christ in Jesus

The winter had set in and it was very cold in the city of Gwalior, where I was born through the grace of Shivgoraksha Babaji. It was a winter's evening of January 1975. My wife was to give birth to my second son

Rudra, and had gone to our family gynecologist. I was relaxed and went to sleep.

At about 10 p.m., I had a wonderful experience, a dream where I saw Jesus The Christ talking to his disciples amongst whom I was seated. He came up to me, smiled, and said, "Keep the good work going, the effort of bringing humanity together as one religion, one Consciousness." Saying this he gently laid his hand upon my forehead and blessed me.

I was aware I was dreaming and told Christ that, "Is this all I'm worth that you should bless me in a dream? Please let this blessing be a reality." After some time my dream came to an end. I opened my eyes and to my utter surprise…the hand that blessed me in my dream was still on my forehead. I broke into a sweat and didn't know what to say; neither did this Divine figure talk. His features were chiseled, a sharp long nose, deep-set brown eyes with a Divine light radiating from them. His eyes spoke as if to say, "Come, I'll show you the way." His hair was dark brown and a little wavy, which matched his wheatish golden complexion. At first I mistook him for an Indian person of royal descent, the great King Vikramaditya.

Later, I noticed his mellow loving appearance. His aura filled my heart with rose and daffodil love. He was dressed in a Judaic Palestinian dress, his hands were as warm as his smile. In silence he blessed me with those flesh and blood hands on my head. I was beside myself and couldn't contain my love for him. Fully awake, I tried to move but was transfixed to my bed. My body had waves of energy flowing through it.

Then the Divine body of Christ in Jesus began dissolving before my eyes till he was gone. The visitation was over all of a sudden and it forged a *karmic* bond between him and the me of my past life. My memory of a past life was renewed, where I had met him in the Himalayas in the *ashram* of a Nath Yogi. I was not able to know the great *yogi*, but it was definite that Jesus learned *Nath Yoga* at this *ashram*. Elsewhere in this book, I have mentioned the name of Jesus' Nath guru of whom I came to know much later.

Divine Mother Durga Experience

In 1978, during the nine sacred days of *Durga Puja*, my family set out for the town of Tulsapur in the state of Maharastra. Tulsapur is the famous place where the Goddess Mahishasur Mardini (Durga) appeared in physical form to the great Marattha warrior King Shivaji and gave him her sword to protect the righteous, destroy the evil, and to establish *dharma* and stability in the land. It was to this very place that we went to seek the blessings of the Divine Mother.

As we reached the place, it was very crowded with hawkers and little shops selling small trinkets and silverware relating to Durga. I very rarely visited public temples and was quite disillusioned with what I saw; the afternoon heat, the noise, the jostling crowd. I prayed to the Mother within me to enable me to find a quiet place in which to meditate away from the noisy crowd. Shivangani, my wife, was with me, and being an ardent Durga devotee was excited for the *dharshan*. So we walked on through the crowd in the heat, with Shivraj, my elder son, on my shoulder while, Rudra, the younger, catching Shivangani's little finger and running along crying, because he was too lazy to walk and wanted her to carry him.

When we reached the temple, I told her not to mention that she was related to the royal family of Shivaji. If she did then a huge ceremony and a big prayer would start, and we would not be able to meditate or do our *Shiva-Shakti Kriya Yoga* practice. As we waited outside the portals of the temple gate, I prayed to the mother, "Like the great Shivaji saw you in person, Oh Mother, can we also see you? Give us a sign, Oh Divine Mother, for we truly yearn to be blessed by Thy presence." As the intensity of my prayer grew, the heat also grew. We were being bothered by flies, but somehow I was becoming transfixed onto the image of the Divine Goddess. Then suddenly a temple priest rushed up to us and said, "Hurry! You are blessed, for you shall get a vision of the Divine Mother."

So he ushered us in through the back door, into the sanctum sanctorium, and there we beheld a great scene. The *Devi's* golden crown, studded with jewels was taken off along with her jewelry and we saw that the true stone image of the Goddess looked nothing like what it did when decorated with all her (*alankar*) jewelry. Then they bathed the Goddess with curds and honey and incense and rosewater. She was astride the lion, holding with her left hand the hair of the demon of negativity and darkness, *Mahishasur*. In her right hand was the divine trident, which pierced his throat of ignorance. After the great bath they adorned her again. All this was done while the curtains were closed to the public. We were special invitees to this event. It was wonderful, but I prayed more passionately in my heart, "Oh, Mother we want a personal divine presence of yours. I'm sure you are not merely a stone image, but a divine and living truth, cosmic as well as personal." And so we left the sanctum and from the back of the temple we walked down the hill to the other side, to a small hamlet.

On another hillock there was yet another temple where they said the Mother went to play the dice of destiny with her celestial angels and a manifestation of Shiva. There I meditated for some time until it was night. We were returning to the temple of the Goddess Bhavani, as she is known in Maharastra. In the dark somebody shouted from atop the hill, "Come on, it's time." I was walking up the hill with Shivraj on my shoulder and shouted back, "I'm coming." This was repeated thrice. Then Shivangani told me that call was for the *Devi* and not for me because it was time to do *aarti* to her (the waving of lights as a sacred gesture of adoration invoking her spirit to bless us). We reached in time for the *aarti* and before it began the conch was blown for purification of the atmosphere around the vicinity. The waving of lights and the showering of flowers began as well. I was transfixed and temporarily became all Consciousness.

Suddenly there emerged from the portals of the sanctum sanctorium two divine ladies dressed in deep green *Kashta saris* (a typical style of Indian dressing with the *sari* separating both legs to enable the woman to ride astride a horse). One of them was about sixty years of age and the other one was eighteen. The whole temple was transformed into a supernal light. My body became light, the floor became light, and the walls became light. The people around me were also weightless and light. Although my eyes were transfixed at the portals, I tried to look at the elderly figure of this Divine Being but my head automatically bowed before the gravity of her Person. I was definitely not hallucinating and was in my fully aware state. Still focusing my mind on the image of the Goddess, the younger of these two figures knew I had not caught the Essence. As I stood with folded arms, she swiftly walked up to me and scratched my forearm, which electrified my whole person. In a flash I saw the sixty year old Being as the Goddess Durga and the eighteen year old as her celestial assistant. Lo and behold! Before my very eyes was the Divine Goddess of Tulsapur. She was the same one who gave the sword to the ancestor of my wife, the great warrior King Shivaji. I couldn't believe my eyes. I saw her, Shivangani saw her, Shivraj saw her and the little Rudra saw her too. We were so blessed.

I know that words are inadequate and insipid to describe the thrill that we felt in our hearts to behold the Divine *Kundalini* in flesh and blood form. Oh my God! What had we done to deserve this? God only knows. This was another awakening to a deeper layer of *Kundalini* which enabled all of us to progress more deeply in our spiritual practices and meditations. All glory be to Thee, Oh Mother.

> *The intake of my every breath*
> *I drink as amrit of Thy Love*
> *And let that nectar mix*
> *In every atom of my blood*

In giving out my breath
I sacrifice my All to Thee
My health, my happiness, my prana
All at Thy Lotus Feet

Oh Divine Mother what can I say? Yet these words rose spontaneously from my heart. No head involved at all. There is no need for the head when you meet the "Heart of the Universe". All I knew was that I was overwhelmed beyond words.

Meditating with Shiva Bala Yogi

I think it was in 1977 that the great Shiva Bala Yogi visited Agra, the city of the Taj Mahal. He came from his *ashram* located in the town of Adivurpapetta near Bangalore and was the honored Guru of his highness of Badhavar the King of the Rajput clan of the Badhorias. His fingers were locked for twelve years during his states of *samadhi*. They say that they needed surgical intervention to separate them.

I was in Gwalior at the time, a town 70 miles to the south of Agra. So my friend, Om Prakash, and I left for Agra that evening. We rested the night in a modest motel, rose early, freshened up and meditated. At 9 o'clock, we rode to the destination in a hackney coach drawn by a horse so underfed and slow that I got the urge to put the horse in the coach and pull it myself. Om Prakash looked at me and we both agreed that at the rate we were moving, we'd reach in the night. But we eventually arrived at 10 am, sooner than expected.

A large congregation of about two thousand people had flocked there to receive the blessings of this Divine Yogi. He was still and seated in lotus posture under a *shamiana* (open tent). We went and seated ourselves comfortably at a distance. Before I knew what was on the agenda, I soon went into a deep trance-like state. Although seeing the people around me, I was aloof. Although hearing their voices, all was a silence within me. This was due to my past *samskaras* connected with Shiva Bala Yogi. As my consciousness associated and familiarized with his wonderful *avasta* (his yogic state of consciousness) I could discern certain past life connections and similarities in *sadhana*.

In the inner circles it is whispered that he is the great Yogi Sri Chandra reincarnated—to this I must agree. Another factor was that Yogi Sri Chandra was considered to be a blessing given to Guru Nanak (the founder of the Sikh religion) by Shiva Goraksha Babaji. Some yogis went on to say that Sri Chandra was an *avatar* of Gorakshanath. My sense of knowingness harmonized with this fact, which may have also been experienced by other *yogis* and Masters. Then all of a sudden he flashed into my mind's eye, flowing and glowing—all smiles. His form changed to Sri Chandra and then he became the formless splendor. My own state of awareness expanded further into my own trueness. My eyes were open and unblinking while my mind was gone and my body rooted to the floor. Mine was the outward gaze with all attention to the inward Soul Consciousness. This was the yogic state called the *shambhave*. This *shambave mudra* was due to my past yogic practices and also due to the blessings of this yogi par excellence who boosted my evolutionary process by awakening me into this *avasta* state.

The *shambhave* is the outward gaze with inward meditation (*dhyana*). The outward gaze looks through the distractions of *maya* into the abyss of nothingness while the inner mind is frozen and transmuted to the Soul Consciousness. Oh *shambhave mudra!* the great seal signifying liberation, all salutations to thee. Although far off, I felt his direct communion—such was the affiliation of being yogis of past lives.

Then Shiva Bala Yogi did something unexpected. He summoned effortlessly by yogic will three boys who were creating a nuisance in the crowd. First their tongues were shut, their bodies transfixed, and then suddenly as though on wheels they slid smoothly on their buttocks in the presence of the great yogi. He did nothing and these mischievous boys who tried to disrupt the *satsang* were soon rolling on the floor crying in pain. This was a natural reaction to their own foul deeds. For in the presence of a realized master of *avataric* stature, one's *karmic* action brings about an immediate, just reaction.

Next Shiva Bala Yogi went into a splendid state of *nirvikalpa samadhi*. He carried with him in his magnetic aura the whole congregation. Each one of us gathered there experienced, according to our past inclinations, a devotional or meditative trance state. We were all bound in a profound state of peace and bliss. Such was the majestic bliss and peace of this monumental yogi. My friend, Om Prakash was in his own state of devotion and I was in my own *avasta*. How time flew by, we had no clue. The others had left and dispersed, some for lunch and some for home.

In the evening I was able to meet him and he was very happy to see me. I instantly knew it was a past life association with him. Then he called me and signaled an okay and a bravo for the good work of yoga that I was doing. He blessed me with an electric touch; an uncanny current passed through my body as he placed his hands on my head. I felt within myself that I was a different man, more confident to spread *Kriya Yoga* with a new zest. *Om Nama Shivaya.*

Meeting the Lion of Judah, Haile Selassie

It was a bleak Autumn morning in London. I had just gotten out of my routine meditation, when all of a sudden, some friends of my host visited. They were very excited and told us that his Majesty, the Emperor of Ethiopia had heard of my experiential Yoga teaching and had expressed a desire to see me, a yogi from India. Haile Selassie (Thrice Great) from the house of Shewa, was also called the "Conquering Lion of Judah", the same title held by King David in the Bible. He was 225th in descent from the line of King Solomon.

Soon, we were driving along in my disciple's Austin Cambridge. Our guides, who had established contacts with the house of Ethiopia, were very happy to be party to this great meeting. I was told to keep this meeting a secret because His Majesty was a guest of the Royal family of England and, for all practical purposes to the African and Ras Tafarian religious communities, he was thought to have left his bodily abode in 1975. However, this was untrue, as I recall meeting with him seven years later in 1982.

Our guides took us to a residence on Great Portland street. We stopped the car and entered a mansion-like home. There were two robust and ruddy men, all smiles, sitting at the reception - Scotland Yard detectives, I presumed. My guess was right, as they simply told us who they were, when we introduced ourselves. He was obviously given the highest security of the land, since the king was a guest of the now late Queen Mary.

The gentlemen led us up a broad red carpeted stairway to a simple but tastefully decorated parlor with soft green furniture and carpet. "The green room of the palace," I said to myself. I was used to all these green and pink rooms which were there at our own house in India. The butler came and asked us if we would like something to drink, but we declined.

We waited for Haile Selassie, the King about whom my grandfather had told me many stories. It is said that Haile Selassie was a visiting board member of the League of Nations. This was the international organization before the United Nations had formed. During an international meeting, a miscreant drew a pistol to shoot the King. He did not move but steadily looked the murderer directly in the eyes. Consequently, the man dropped his pistol and was led away by the security guards.

After about a twenty-minute wait, his Majesty, the King entered. We all stood up and bowed. He responded to our bows and bade us to sit down. He was accompanied by his grandson, a very impressive person, seven feet tall and about twenty-five years of age. He was introduced to us as Prince Jacob, pronounced *Ya-kub* as in Hebrew. He had completed his military studies in the National Defense Academy in Pune, my hometown in India.

When pleasantries had been exchanged, cakes and pastries eaten, his Majesty arose and so did we all, according to the royal protocol. He went into his inner chamber and requested me to follow. As we sat opposite one another, I had the opportunity to have a deeper look at him. He was about ninety years of age. His eyes were aglow with the experience of life. His stoic head was held steady on his sturdy shoulders. His hair was curly and white as snow. When I peered into his heart I saw his truly majestic and lion soul. Oh, what a sight! What a man! "Truly great men do not have to show what they are. They are what they are!" I thought. I was 38 years of age then.

He asked me if I could perform a *havan*, a fire ceremony, for him and his family. I consented to do so but told him of the smoke, which may cause the fire alarm to go off. He made all the arrangements and also informed the Scotland Yard security guards. And so we got under way preparing for the sacred fire ceremony.

I told the King that in ancient times, around 7000 BC, a great king from India called Mahan Data had performed a stupendous *havan* in the Congo basin in Africa. This was mentioned in the *Puranas*. Of course it's a metaphorical saying that the sand in many parts of the Congo resembles holy ash. However, it is interesting to note that it does appear that that sand is the remnant of an ancient fire ceremony.

He showed a great interest in ancient history and told me that was trade via the Silk Road between Ethiopia and India before Cleopatra's time. It was during the time of the Queen Sheba of Ethiopia that Africa learned a lot of the spiritual lore and spiritual techniques from India. This was later passed on from Ethiopia to the Egyptians. I was deeply intrigued to hear this from the King who himself was a deeply spiritual and divine Soul. In India we call such a Soul a *Mahatma* or a "Great-Soul" like Mahatma Gandhi. Such Souls visit our earth rarely.

Many interesting things I learned that day from this great King Sage who reminded me of the ancient King Janaka of the Ramayana. I also told him that Bhima, the Pandava Prince and cousin of Lord Krishna had married a girl called Hedamba from Ethiopia.

As we talked all the preparations for the fire ceremony were made: the clarified butter, the rice, *etc*. I then proceeded to perform the *havan* for the welfare of humanity and for spiritual progress to all. The sacred flames of the fire ceremony danced to the chanting of *mantras*. All those present were engulfed in the holy ambiance as we rejoiced in the Spirit of the Lord.

After this sacred ceremony was over, his Majesty was very touched. He and the Queen then showed me what they needed to show me. As I passed through their bed chamber I looked at him and his majestic bed. I thought it to be made of platinum or white gold but did not ask him. The royal bed was so huge with its curtains that I mistook it for another small chamber.

Upon his showing an interest in the science of Yoga, I gave to him the yogic *Hamsa* breathing technique, which he practiced successfully. Six months later, he telephoned me in India and told me of the spiritual well-being and sound sleep he was able to have after practicing the technique.

Meeting Ambha Baba – The Miracle Worker

It was during 1978, in the town of Gwalior that I first came across
Ambha Baba, named after the village he came from. I was sitting at
Deshraj Singh Chauhan's place, a very dear friend of my father. Sitting
there was also a tall bald man with a radiant face and eyes that looked
out into the nowhere. Not only was he not all there, but I observed he
was blind too. This, however, did not seem to be a handicap in his
moving around or doing his daily chores. I was about thirty plus years
old then and was well established in my meditation. My spiritual practice
(*sadhana*) had developed a definite clairvoyance in me. As I looked
at the saint, I was able to perceive that he had the *siddhi* of the
nineteenth of the 52 *Veers*. Without hesitation, I asked the *baba* if he
had the *siddhi* of the nineteenth *Veer*. He smiled and retorted, "You
are mischievous aren't you? Prying into my astral."

However, he expressed a desire to visit my ancestral home,
which I immediately fulfilled. My father Deshraj Singh, my wife
Shivangini and my two sons, Shivraj and Rudra, were all present.
Knowing that Ambha Baba possessed *siddhis*, we requested him to
bless our home and give us an experience of his *siddhis*. He consented
and asked us for a clean bed sheet. Then he went into my bathroom,
bathed and came out with only the washed bed sheet wrapped around
him. I led the blind baba into my meditation room. On sitting there for
sometime, he uttered the names of Shiva-Goraksha-Babaji, Lahiri
Mahasaya, Sri Yukteswar and all the gods and godessess of my wife's
puja. He *pranamed* (joined his hands and bowed) and said that the
room was too powerful for him to perform his miracles. I had noticed
that in spite of his blindness, he was able to see the exact photos of the
gurus on the wall. This gave me to know that he was a man of inner
understanding, with the divine eye.

He came out into the living room and asked for a silver tray
and a lamp to be lit. We did that, and as we sat around the table, he
asked us what we would like to eat. Shivraj at once jumped at the

chance and asked for *pedas* (an Indian sweet) and Rudra asked for grapes. The Saint opened the bed sheet, which covered him and showed us his bare body, then put his hands over the silver tray and meditated. We all watched with bated breath, and Deshraj Bhaisaab, my father, observed with scientific attitude. We believed but just wanted to make sure this was not some trick or sleight of the hand.

Then suddenly, before our open eyes, there was a sound and the *peda* sweets hit the bottom of the saint's hands and fell onto the tray quite fresh. We all touched the sweetmeats to see if they were real. Next came the black grapes called *anabshahi*, and then the green grapes called "Seedless Thompson." Although I was firmly set upon the path of Self-Realization and God alone, I was nonetheless overcome by intrigue, wanting to know more about the wonders of God and the miracles of Nature. This marvelous exhibition of miracles went on till the table looked rich with food. I ordered a rare Bengal rice called *Ananda Bhoga*, which is well known for its long grain and delightful flavor. Lo and behold! It was there on the table along with biscuits, cake and fruit. A feast fit for the eyes and the belly of a king. Nothing was wanting. All that was asked for had been materialized from thin air.

This was no trick but a genuine display of the *siddhi* of this saint. So I thought that it could perhaps have been a formation of an ectoplasmic substance at the palm of his hands, which he later converted by his will to any desired fruit or edible commodity. It could have been a direct transference of goods from the relevant shops or orchards or a direct *siddhi*, where he materialized by *Iccha Shakti* the foods we asked for. But all this is speculation. The important fact was that the Saint himself did not give much importance to his *siddhis*. He was not stuck in his miracles, but occasionally showed them to demonstrate their worthlessness in comparison to the ultimate and true *siddhi*, which he said was the realization of God!

Later, when everyone had gone, he called me aside and putting his arms around my shoulders said, "You know my son, all this pomp and show is a game of *maya* and does not last. The only true *siddhi* is the *siddhi* of God, all else is illusion. Don't be impressed with this glitter of showmanship. It shall all melt in the magic dream. Only the Lord shall last forever. You are on the true path. Keep it up and spread God's work in the world. Teach Yoga. It is the supreme path of liberation." Saying this, he left my ancestral home, leaving behind his goodwill and blessings to us all.

King Barthahari Nath of Ujjain

One day during my winter vacations, I took the night bus and traveled to Ujjain. The whole night I meditated in the bus alternating it with the *Om Namah Shivaya japa*. During my travel in the bus I was explaining to a friend of mine called Mulik how fortunate aspiring yogis were and how a certain yogi saw with his very own eyes the majestic figure of the King of Ujjain, called Raja Barthahari. The morning twilight blushed the sky as the first rays of the Sun were beginning to appear upon the horizon. I went on in the meantime with my story, describing the face and beard of Barthahari Nath, who was a direct disciple of the deathless Shiva-Gorakshanath. I told my friend that a yogi had seen the great Nath on these very roads of Ujjain in the early hours of the dawn.

The bus stopped, we got down and started walking on the road, which was at least sixty feet wide. I continued talking, saying, "Barthahari Nath was six foot six inches tall with white dreadlocks tied up like a temple dome on the top of his head, inviting the crescent moon to settle on top of it, making him appear like the veritable Shiva. But he had a very dull colored torn gunny sack cloth that covered his body. Around the gunny sack was a big red sash and to it was tied a huge bell which hit his right and left thigh as he majestically walked along these very roads. Wasn't he fortunate?" I asked my friend. "And the bell, as it hit each thigh, made the sound of 'clang-clang, clang-

clang.'" Lo and behold, as I lifted my gaze, to the other side of the road I heard the sound of bells, "clang-clang, clang-clang." I was wonder-struck to see the image of Raja Barthahari exactly as I had described it to my friend Mulik. My eyes were transfixed on him. My feet were rooted to the ground.

In the early hours with the traffic gently flowing by, I stretched my hands back to bring this wondrous sight to Mulik's notice. But he was nowhere to be found or seen. I tried to surge forward across the road and clasp his feet in my arms, but that majestic figure transfixed me with a gaze and rooted me to the ground. He was a tall, six and a half foot man with the (*jatta*) matted dreadlocks crowning his head wearing a gunnysack garment with a red sash as his belt and the bell making the sound so typical of the Nath Yogi. He was not wearing the *arband nag* black belts of wool as he is usually depicted in pictures drawn in Maharashtra. *Yogis* usually tie the belts, also called *Bhairava Bana*, when they go begging for alms or during their meditation. What I had described to my friend with such sincerity and wanted to see myself, I saw instantly on the same road, which the former yogi had seen. This was indeed a great fortune and blessing for me.

And later on as I meditated that night by the Shipra river, haunted with the romantic tales of the legendary Nath Yogis, before my mind's eye again came this majestic Yogi King, Barthahari, with black belts, who transformed himself into the smiling Lahiri Mahasaya, the *Kriya Yoga* Master. With him also I had the vision of the Master Kabir who smilingly transformed himself into the great Sai Baba of Shirdi. And both in unison said, "*Alakh Gorakhia Babaji. Alakh Gorakhia Babaji.*" On reflection, I realized as an afterthought, in deep meditations that Barthahari had been taken for his mission and penances by Gorakshanath when his queen the Maharani Pingala died, and he had left with a heavy heart.

Gorakshanath saw to it that his desire for a grand palace and the householder wife were preserved in his causal body, so that in a later incarnation Babaji could pull this lofty soul down, get him married to the Divine Kashi Moni. Then after he became a householder yogi as Lahiri Mahasaya, Babaji fulfilled the purposefully kept desire of seeing the grandest palace a mortal could ever imagine. If Babaji had not kept this desire preserved in the mind of the King Barthahari, nobody could ever make such a lofty Soul as Yogavatar Lahiri Mahasaya, incarnate into the haunts of mortal man. No power in the world could keep Lahiri Mahasaya away from his guru Gorakshanath Babaji, the *Mahavatar*. So blessed be Babaji Goraksha and blessed be the King Barthahari Nath who incarnated as the householder Yogavatar, Lahiri Mahasaya, for the salvation of the world.

This vision of mine goes to show that such great Divine Masters as the King Barthahari Nath, Kabir and Lahiri Mahasaya are one at the highest Divine level of *avataric* Consciousness. That is, the *nirvanic* Consciousness of Lahiri Mahasaya and Kabir are also One. These bodies are a mere choosing of a garment for a particular divine mission on this terrestrial world.

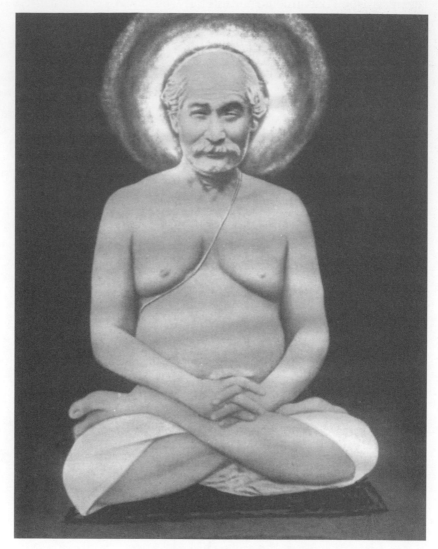

Yoga Avatar Lahiri Mahasaya
*in his former life was Mahayogi Kabir, and the life before that
was Yogiraj Bhartarinath. In all three incarnations he was
a direct disciple initiated into Kriya-Raj Yoga
by Shiva Goraksha Babaji.*

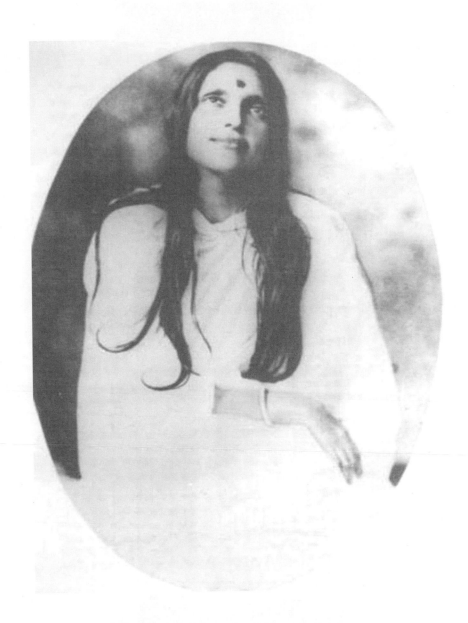

*Anandamayi Ma, who blessed Siddhanath
with spiritual experiences & graced him to
spread Babaji's Kriya Yoga the world over*

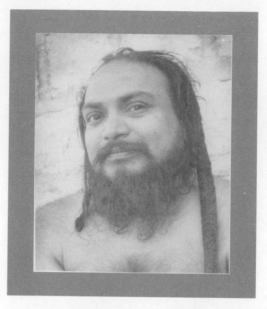

*Shiva Bala Yogi, an incarnation of Mahayogi Shri Chandra
the son of Guru Nanak Deva. Shri Chandra was initiated by
the Divine Shiva Goraksha Babaji*

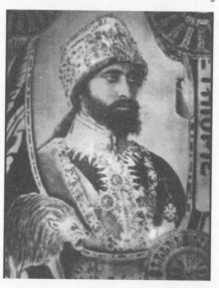

*Emperor of Ethiopia Haile Selassie descendant of
the family lineage of King Solomon and his wife Queen of Shiba*

CHAPTER 7

ON HEALING AND BEING HEALED
The Casting Out of Evil Spirits

It was the second week after the incident at Saundha of which I have related in Chapter Four, that I went down to a small village, the name of which I no longer remember. It was not Saundha, it was some other village. The people of the village said that there was some lady who had had a vision of the sage Dattatreya by an Avadumbar tree, and she was able to foretell events, cure people, and exorcise evil spirits. So it was that later, a temple was built there in honor of Dattatreya. I went there and thought that I would visit the temple and see what was going on. So in the evening, I trudged along with the setting sun. I set off for the other village. The only means of transport was by foot. So, like in Rajasthan, where you see little boys kicking up the dust, that's exactly what I was doing. I was idling my time kicking up the dust. It was not sand, but mud.

The sun was setting as I was going along in the middle of the road between the passing sheep. My hair and the sheep's hair became orange. We were all dyed by the color of the sun. A voice came to me from within, "Do not go to this village. It will turn against you. But, if you do go, do not turn back. Return victorious." I said to myself that I would go on, since I had set my foot upon the given path. Patting and petting the wool on the sheep backs, I walked and walked and walked.

When I reached my destination, I saw a peculiar, strange aura. This I sensed was a very strange place. Then I went to the Avadumbar tree, did my *pranam* and sat down. There was a young, pretty lady who was sitting there and everyone was touching her feet. I went up to her, but she got up and touched my feet as I did *pranam*. She must have seen or had psychic vision as to who I was. At that time, I myself was unaware of my own spiritual state. I sat down and asked her who she was. She replied, "I'm so and so and I'm from a Gorpade family."

After some time, I got up and walked a little and noticed that there was an *aarti* going on. About a hundred people had gathered around the tree when it started. Suddenly I heard a noise as I was praying. Women then appeared with their hair hanging loose and the men began swaying and chanting. On the ground was a person turning somersaults. It appeared to me that this entire village was possessed of evil spirits. I thought to myself, "Where have I landed myself?" Over 300 people were possessed with spirits of sorts. I prayed, "Oh Lord, what sort of an ordeal is this? All these spirits will come onto me and I'll have a whole village of spirits in me." I laughed for I was well fortified with the protection and power of Lord Shiva.

Why do these spirits come? They come because they are dissatisfied souls with unfulfilled desires. To fulfill their desires, they enter the human body and through the human body they fulfill their desires. Spirits often ask for *jalebee*, a circular Indian sweet. Actually, they have no tongue, no means to fulfill their desires. If they want a new shirt, through you they will wear a new shirt or wear a new *sari*, and in that way they will enjoy themselves. They will be happy in it. And then they will leave. That is the first reason. The second reason is in continuity with the first reason. Many people are killed in accidents, which is called premature death or *akaal mrityu*. So they have to mark time in limbo or *bardo*, the etheric and astral regions, until their original death time comes, at which time they are naturally released from their *bardo* state. This is also called *Bhuva Loka* (astral plane) or *Narka Lok*, which are Nether regions of darkness and despair.

In Christian terms, it is a hell of a place. For those who have this type of death, their physical body dies, but their emotional being and unfulfilled desires are still vibrant. So in order to fulfill them, they seek an entry into any human being who has a weak astral body. They enter into the consciousness of a person through the central nervous system and autonomous nervous system. This is how they control the body. They thereby fulfill their desires, whatever they may be.

Saint Zanyabai's good spirit entered the girl's body in the village of Vrideshwar. It was to cure her nervous debility. That person was suffering from a nervous disorder and a slightly demented state, which could be healed. So therefore, that spirit came to infuse the flow of nervous energy in the brain so that her thinking could be brought into proportion. That good spirit came for a good cause.

But, there are bad spirits that enter bodies too. They ravage it and put it to great task. These spirits are of a dream state, a laughing state, a crying state, and all sorts of shades and grades of spirits. It's all psychicism. Spiritual people don't usually involve themselves in this sphere of the subject, even if they come across it like I did. They steer clear of it. If they are strong enough, they deal with those spirits without forgetting their goal of merging their individual with Divine Consciousness. These spirits are *bardo* experiences of which the Tibetans make much ado. These experiences are to be had, learnt, and then let go of. The *yogi* treats the experiences of *bardo-thol* and death with impunity. Overriding death, he fearlessly strives only for the clear light of *prajna* and *samadhi*.

To continue with the experience at this village, I just went near those possessed people who then said, "Don't burn us. We will go out". So I asked them when they would go out. "On the full moon," they replied. The full moon was a week from that day, so I said, "If I show you the full moon now, will you go out?" They agreed. So I caught one person by his hair and hit his head with mine. He jumped up and fell on the floor. After he came to his normal self, I asked him if he had seen the full moon. He replied that he had but added that he had also seen spots and starry things. I then told him that everyone sees stars when hit on the head. I said, "That is a common phenomenon, but did you see the moon?" He replied, "I saw the moon very clearly." I asked, "Are you going?" He said, "Give me permission to go and don't burn me." Saying this, he left the body he possessed as it fell to the floor with a thud. Then I went on exorcising the other spirits. Some challenged me and said, "This is the place of Dattatreya. Where have you come from?" I answered, "I have come from the place of Mahadeva, Lord Shiva." "Oh," they said, "that's okay."

Another person was somersaulting on the ground all day long. I said to him, "From now on, you don't somersault. Just sit down and the spirit will go." I tapped him on the back, ran my hand along his spine and in the evening, when the *aarti*, the sacred waving of *niranjana* wick lamps was being done, he saw me. He was about to somersault, but he caught my eye and didn't. So after exorcising the spirits, at night we were given our places and we rested.

The huts were small with bare floors and nothing else. The spirits were exorcised from the huts, but there was still quite a stench in the whole area because the spirits sometimes caused the possessed bodies to urinate in their huts. The bad ones leave their odor and the good ones their fragrance, but in such places the good astral spirits do not come very often. As I lay down in the night amongst the people possessed, I thought to myself that I must have created some strange *karma* in my past life to be put in such a weird situation. Strangely, I seemed to be quite at home with it.

The next morning, the people came and said, "Oh, the village chief is calling you." They said, "Look, we hear you have been exorcising spirits in the town." They came to me and took me before the village chief Patil, who asked, "Do you think that you are greater than Dattatreya? That you come to this place and you have the audacity to exorcise spirits?" There was a committee of people sitting there. That night there was also a marriage going on, and a fire was lit upon which was being cooked a huge dish of rice called *pullava*. This is a common dish, which is eaten by all people during marriages in India.

I replied, "No, I don't think anything. I had just come to this town to pay my respects to the Dattatreya. As I saw some people suffering in their plight of being possessed, I relieved them from that state." They said, "No, no, you are telling a lie. You have come to show your arrogance as a yogi. We have seen many such yogis, and you are all false yogis." I answered, "All right, if you say so. But go and see the results. See the people who have been exorcised, see who has the spirit in them. I am not claiming anything. I took the *darshan* of Dattatreya. I went to that lady. I acknowledged what she had seen. That was it. I follow the Nath Yogi's tradition and I came from Shiva's temple in yonder village."

They said, "No, we have seen many such people. You come here and you want to make money by trying to show that you are somebody special." I said, "I have no such thing in mind, and please don't worry me too much because I have had enough. I am tired now. I am going without food for so many days. Please don't worry me."

They asked, "Where do you come from?" I said, "I'm coming from Mahadev, the Ancient of Days, Lord Shiva. I have just come for my *bhakti*." I was in a very devotional state and tears flowed down my cheeks, and these people kept disparaging me. I said, "Okay, I can go away tomorrow. I have no need to be here. I have just come here because I wanted to serve you all." They retorted, "Oh, we don't need that. Dattatreya is there for us."

One man said, "This yogi has an evil eye on that girl over there." I don't know what happened next. Such a roar came out of me, "AAAAAAH! *Alak Niranjan*! Don't you dare to say that! The place will lose its spirituality. My God!" And they were stunned! "There will be no place here, because it is my purity of intention versus your false allegations. If I am false, burn me in hell, but if you are false, nothing will happen to you because you have a loose tongue and you don't know who you are talking to." And then, I shoved my foot into the burning fire. "Here!" And then I put my hand inside. "You are idiots! You do not know who is coming." And then I admonished them in the village language. My hand was in the fire and they ran and pulled my hand out of the fire. There was nothing, no burn marks. They begged, "Swami Maharaj, please forgive us, we didn't know who you were." My shout was so loud, it was like the roar of a lion, that the village music stopped. The marriage ceremony stopped. They said, "We are doing the wrong thing. We challenged this yogi. He is one of the Nath Yogis."

Then another *yogi* came and he said, "Today you have won and I have lost." I replied, "I have nothing to win or lose." He said, "No, but I have seen. I was ahead of you in *sadhana*, but when you did this, and you gave this roar, I realized that the work is to be handed over to you. You shall be world famous. You shall go to America, Europe and all these places and the whole world will listen to what you have to say. But your family members will not listen to you. They will not listen to that extent of in-depth *sadhana*. They will start listening later, for the people at home are the last to acknowledge and listen. As far as the evolution of human consciousness goes, I would be honored to be a servant of humanity as my larger Self. When you gave that shout and that roar, in that I saw the power of Shiva-Goraksha-Babaji. It was a supreme shout. In that shout your whole history, your whole character, your past, present and future were revealed."

I said, "I don't know what you are trying to say. Why are you praising me? I am not concerned about this. I am concerned about the here and now. I have come here. I have done my work and now I am going." "No, no, don't go. We have made a mistake," said the people of the *panchayat* and then the elders of the village realized their mistake. I said, "Nothing doing, I am not going to wait here." But they insisted and made me wait. They apologized and asked me to stay for the *aarti* on the next day.

I slept there that night and in the morning I got up, opened my door and found all the village spirits were awake. There was the sunrise silhouette of one naked person running in the twilight with his *lota*, that is, vessel of water, and racing to the toilet before the spirit possessed his body. It was a beautiful scene. Then everybody got up and the activity of the devil village, the ghost village, started. I was swayed with the spirits. It was very enjoyable, to sway, being possessed. They were also possessed. They were possessed by spirits and I was possessed by the Divine Spirit.

This was a past life recapitulation when I went to exorcise spirits, cured and healed people. I am done with this healing and curing now. According to Shiva-Goraksha-Babaji, my work is to give the Here Now state and get people to the clear light, not to tamper with the *bardo-thol*, that is, the dream state, the psychic state, and the astral state, which my teachings have nothing to do with. I penetrate through these astral and psychic phenomena to get to the clear light, the *prajna*. The *yogis* of India have caught the *bardo* experiences by the forelocks and thrown them out of their lives. They also taught the Tibetan and Buddhist yogis and ascetics to do the same and focus on the Divine, and not get caught up in astral *maya* and the *tantric* ways.

In the morning it was time for the *aarti*. The *aarti* was sung and the spirits that had been exorcised by me had been noticed by the village chief who was in charge. He saw exactly who was not possessed. They did not show any sign of swaying or moving. I told him it was not me but by the grace of Shiva-Goraksha-Babaji and of Dattatreya that this has happened. Then I thanked them for their hospitality and advised them to beware next time and not to open their mouths unnecessarily. They must see which yogi comes to them, and learn from him. When a yogi comes and wants to offer you something, you must not miss the opportunity. I bade them farewell and left the village.

After this I rested, because I was quite exhausted with 300 spirits hovering around me and trying to vampire on my spiritual energy. I must explain here that there are various spiritual and *tantric* feminine energies such as the *dakhinis*, *kakanis*, *hakinis*, and *larkinis etc*. These *shaktis* often help or obstruct a yogi on his spiritual path, depending upon the *yogi*'s individual *karma*. Their main objective is to strengthen the yogi's astral body and mind. By this a *yogi* is prepared to go on to more intensive *sadhana* and higher states of yogic awareness.

I must warn that these astral entities test a person right from the state of sex till one reaches the highest state of meditation. Only when a yogi has crossed the threshold of meditation and entered into the clear light of *samadhi* consciousness is he free from these feminine astral energies. But many a yogi and spiritual devotee have crossed into the higher states, brushing aside these *dakhini* energies. Many have done it in the past and many shall be victorious in the future.

I returned victorious and heard the mystic voice of the *dakhini*, "Yes, I told you the whole village will turn against you and warned you not to go to the village. If you did, you must return victorious. This is a great victory for you." I don't know what she meant by "great victory". Maybe it was some past life *karma* that I had overcome and had nothing to do with now. After this I went back to Vrideswar, to the spiritual pilgrimage center of Mahadeva Shiva.

Surya Yoga: Pranic Healing of Solar Power

All along my yogic journey, as years passed by, I practiced and moved into techniques that were most natural to me. With the grace of Babaji I developed a dynamic process of self-healing. I called it *Otaprot-Surya* meaning osmotic solar healing. It is not possible for me to give the technique in its totality, because of the advanced nature of certain practices. This, of course, renders these techniques impractical for teaching to all people. Hence I had to give a simpler solar self-healing technique to my student-teachers (*Hamsacharyas*).

The *Surya*, solar self-healing techniques are basically purifying and rejuvenating in nature. When you absorb the radiant energy of the spiritual sun, all toxins of the system are flushed out. Every cell in the body is permeated with life giving *prana*. This *prana* is the universal life-force energy that pervades the universe at all levels. Light, heat, gravity, magnetism and cohesion all need *prana* as their motivating life.

Deep rooted syndromes and negative patterns of behavior surface during the practice of solar *pranayam*. But I worked out the breathing techniques so that these negative syndromes would dissolve without creating undue emotional upheaval.

The positive effects of *Surya Kavach* (protective sun-shield) and *Swashan-Jwala* (breath-of-fire) *pranayamas* are self-evident. These healthful patterns of breathing increase your memory recall, enhance concentration and build stamina. The will to achieve one's goal and the courage to cope with the rough and tumble of daily life are the blessings of the radiant life giving sun (*Surya*). When the breath and fire breathing is done with the *Hams-Sa*, it opens up new vistas of consciousness in the brain so necessary for one's spiritual evolution.

Then I found it necessary to develop and give to aspirants and practicing *yogis* a *mudra*—an effective *mudra* whereby the salubrious rays of the sun can enter and heal the body. Remember that the body needs to be a fit temple to enable its divine indweller to evolve. So I developed the *Guru-Shishya Mudra* meaning the Master-Disciple hand posture. I found that when I practice the solar meditation with this *mudra*, a lot more energy flowed into my physical and astral body *chakras*.

The blissful energy descending into the crown *chakra* is ineffable. It is the power and joy of Shiva, the first aspect of the Divine Trinity flowing in. This doesn't always happen. The experience happened to me for the first time in the Himalayas at Rudraprayag. I was basking on the river beach at Koteswar Shiva temple. When I looked at the sun, its magnetic radiance pulled me up, and I saw in the solar orb an image of myself with my hands atop my head. I formed the same *mudra* posture and felt the surge of Shiva's energy. I later called this the "Temple of Humanity" *mudra*. After experiencing the effect of the *mudra*, I was overjoyed with the bounties of the sun and of nature. These verses flowed out in praise of the sun.

Surya Yoga Meditation

I drink oh drink thee Sun of Life
Your roaring radiance rinses me through
Gushing through spine with Sizzling joy
I thy Divinity enjoy!

From thy elysian fountain rays
I drink immortal Pranic Life
Rejuven Body and my mind
Dissolve all worldly woe and strife!

Dancing with thine immortal light
Each cell suffused with joy of Life
I glorify this gift oh Lord
No Emperor ever can afford!

Orange elixirs wine sublime
Flows, glows in every fiber mine
Filling me with thy Bliss sublime
Making me to My Self Divine!

To my simple way of thinking the sun is the one in whom we live and move and have our being. We drink of its life and float in its radiant soup. All human beings are saturated with the life giving essence of the sun. Neither humans nor plants would survive without its light and energy. Therefore the sun (*Surya*) is our immediate *deva* (god) whom we must love, adore and worship every day to lead and guide us to the Supreme Lord God! The virtues of the sun qualify it to be our *deva* and immediate archangel who sustains all life on earth.

The sun gives us knowledge and wisdom, and frees us from ignorance and impenetrable darkness. Therefore we should look up to the sun to guide us from darkness to light. There is a parable that is taught to illustrate how knowledge is used to free us from ignorance. Let us take ignorance as a thorn. One thorn has entered into our foot. Now let us take another thorn, knowledge, to remove the first thorn. When we take out the thorn of ignorance with the help of the thorn of knowledge, we can say that we enter into the realm of death and conquer it. Once we have taken out the troubling thorn, we do not need the thorn that has entered into our foot and we do not need the thorn that we used to remove it. At that time we go beyond both knowledge and ignorance and enter into the light of wisdom.

The Gayatri and the Aditya Surya Mantras

There are two *mantras* which have inspired and transformed my life. In India, these *mantras* are taught to children by their parents. They permeate the fabric of Indian society and form an integral portion of the perennial philosophy of *Sanatana Dharma*.

Gayatri Mantra

Bhur Bhuvaha Svaha
Tat Savitur Varenyam
Bhargo Devasya Dhee Mahe
Dhiyo Yo Naha Prachodayat

We meditate on the supreme
Effulgence of the Divine
Solar Creator that he may
Make us to Ourselves Divine

The *Gayatri* is one of the most sacred *mantras* to *Surya*, the deity of our sun. This is a gift to humanity from Rishi Vishwamitra, who

127

is the seer of the third book of the *Rig Veda*. It expedites one's spiritual evolution and enlightens one's intellect to that effect.

The heroic Vishwamitra is the archetype of the yogic way. He demonstrated the strength and will of the greatest of all solar initiates. He was one of the most excellent of all Vedic *rishis* and yet the most controversial. He began as a great king and warrior who was not from a priestly or *brahmanic* family, but decided to change by his *tapas* (austere practice) from his warrior status to the spiritual status of a seer. This brought him into conflict with the priestly order.

His was the path of a warrior, of discipline and struggle, defeat and victory. He persisted through all difficulties including those created by his own ambition until after a long period of spiritual practice, he ultimately achieved self-realization through his willpower and *tapas*. His path therefore is considered the result more of human effort (*purshartha*) rather than only Divine Grace (*Ishvar Kripa*).

Vishwamitra did not stop at anything. With his indomitable will he overcame all obstacles and even challenged the gods. When he meditated, he created by his *tapas* such an internal fire and heat, that externally its smoke clouds and heat began to threaten the gods in heaven. The demi-gods became jealous of his spiritual prowess so they sent a celestial nymph called Meneka to seduce him and divert him from his intense meditation. So strong was his solar practice that if he had opened his eyes, she would have been burnt to cinders, so Meneka had to approach him from behind. However, Vishwamitra decided that she would be the right mother for a family of kings who would rule the lands, so he accepted a small delay in his austerities for this purpose.

From his union with the celestial maiden was born a beautiful daughter called Shakuntala who eventually became the wife of king Dushyanta. King Bharat, from whom the name of India as Bharat arose was the son of Shakuntala.

The Aditya Surya Mantra
A Solar Incantation

Om Aditya Hridayam Punyam
Sarva Shatru Vinashanam
Jaya Vaham, Japam Nityam
Akshayam Paramam Shivam

Oh Surya purify my heart
Destroy all enemies within and without
I ceaselessly chant thy victorious name
Oh indestructible supreme Sun Shiva!

Aditya Hridayam is a sacred *mantra* in praise of the sun, invoking his blessings to open up the devotee's heart (*hridayam*) to the divine light of the sun. This hymn is part of the sixth part of the epic *Ramayana*, attributed to the *Siddha* sage Valmiki. The *Ramayana* is a tale of the divine hero Rama and his battle to eradicate the darkness of evil and bring justice and light back to the world. The champion of evil was the king of Lanka, called Ravana.

The stage for the hymn is the battlefield, where Rama and Ravana are fighting, being watched by yogic sages and divine light beings. One of the foremost sages watching this epic struggle was Agastya, who noticed that Rama, for all his valor and strength was getting tired, since Ravana was practically invincible and invulnerable to weapons. Immediately seeing the danger to the order of the universe, Agastya approached and initiated Rama into the solar hymn of divine light, the *Aditya Hridayam*.

The sage reminded Rama of the unlimited power and energy of the visible manifestation of the Divine Creator, the *Surya-Aditya*, and the boundless Divine love of *Surya-Mitra*, which enables humanity to call upon this immense reservoir of energy. Renewed by the connection with the sun, Rama acquired the knowledge and strength to continue his battle and eventually defeat Ravana.

It is through this hymn that Rama has taught all humanity that the sun is the manifest divinity, the *pratyaksha daivam*, whom we can see every day and to whom we can show our gratitude and connect with the essential solar energy. Agastya also taught that the sun is the repository of all yogic knowledge, and by forming a relationship with *Surya*, humanity can acquire the means to Self-Realization.

Incident with the Armor of Surya

It was a summer morning in the town of Gwalior, in India. I arose early, bathed and meditated in the salubrious rays of the sun. I did my *Surya Yoga*, the solar healing technique. It involved the *Aditya Hridayam mantra*, dynamic *pranayamas* and a *Surya Kavach*, or protective shield, which I had developed by spreading with my hands the rays of the sun all over the body. It was like applying a sacred balsam or oil all over my body. This made me feel as though a magnetic barrier of light had been formed around me. I felt very energized and fulfilled every time I did this. Ever since my childhood I have been fascinated by the rising and setting sun. In spite of myself, I was drawn to and magnetized by this huge orb of orange elixir, from whose health-giving rays I drank freely.

After my *Surya Yoga* I laid down to read a yoga book. There was a knock on my door and, as I opened it, some friends came and told me that a house belonging to them had been occupied by some miscreants. These illegal squatters refused to leave this small house which was adjacent to an old cinema theatre named "Delight Talkies".

As I went with my friends, they told me that the Judiciary Court had given legal notice to the miscreants to evacuate the house. In spite of this they had refused to obey the court orders, and started pulling strings with influential contacts. Anyhow we approached the new road, as it was called, situated in the local bazaar. We waited for the Court

Nizam, the judicial messenger who was to serve the notice of evacuation. But an hour passed and he did not turn up. Neither did the police who were at standby to ensure a smooth transition. The building had been given to Sadhuram Godarwal, a tailor stitching clothes for the family of a nobleman called Sardar Patankar.

The minutes ticked by and the afternoon sun was beating down upon us. The building to be taken over was in front of me and the Indian sweet shops were behind me. The sweet makers stirred their gigantic frying pans, and the aroma of dairy sweets in the making filled the air. It was time to move in, but God only knew what was in store for us. A huge wrestler joined our group and promised to help us capture the house, which in any case was legally ours. He jumped on a bed in the attempt to climb the back wall. The bed broke and that was the end of his mission. I moved towards the house with Patankar and four others. The hoodlums warned us not to come. "The consequences would be serious," they shouted.

Heedless to their warnings we steadily closed in on the house and then all hell broke loose! There emerged from the parapets of the house and the adjoining theatre scores of people. They began throwing soda water bottles and stones at us. The soda bottles landed and burst all around us. I heard the sweet makers shouting in their open shops. Some had been hit on their heads as the bottles burst. So they pulled their shutters down. Other shops had their showcases and windows broken. A huge crowd of over a thousand people had gathered. Many of the people accompanying me in this righteous action had fled because of injury from the bottles.

The sun beat down on me mercilessly as I stood my ground. Then I saw and felt the strangest experience of my life. Stones and bottles were being deflected as they came within three yards of me. I felt a pneumatic pressure surrounding me. I saw through this pressure of *prana*, a radiance emanating from my body. Dumbfounded with this phenomenon, I was silent within as the storm raged around me.

The people had swelled in numbers, all gathered to see this free show. It became too unreal—a *tamasha*, like a film show. Eventually I single-handedly confronted about twenty people, amidst a barrage of soda bottles and stones being thrown at me. I made a full-on contact with a huge hoodlum. His protruding belly vibrated like jelly and he backed out as I entered the house with Patankar following. When the miscreants saw this, they withdrew, and sent down some screaming women with long fingernails. I did not touch these women because of my principles and the norms of the Indian society. They tried to scratch me first and then my friend, but stopped short. The reason for their sudden change of behavior from screaming cats to docile kittens surprised those very women. "The *Surya*," I thought and then it flashed on me, that my solar meditations had created a magnetic barrier of light around me. This *pranic* light was the cause of my protection during the whole incident.

So we backed out of the house onto the road and into the sweltering heat. As soon as I was on the road, the barrage of stones and old soda bottles began again. There is a marble stuck in the neck of these old soda bottles, and if shaken well and thrown, they exploded onto whatever they are thrown at. I was parched and badly needed a drink. Suddenly a Coca-Cola bottle was thrown at me. I caught it, opened it with my teeth and drunk the cola. Cool and soothing it was, my thirst quenched, I was about to throw the bottle back but my Self made me roll it back. This led to a lot of embarrassment to the person who had attacked me because I gave him love in return.

Too much time was being spent. I had to take possession of the building at any cost. I had given Patankar my word. So the next time I advanced, I was met by an angry fellow with a steel rod in his hands. He was threatening. His hands with the raised steel bar remained raised in the air. He was glued and couldn't move. My eyes were transfixed to his. Then Patankar and my friend pulled me off the stairs of the house. The moment I was away down came the steel bar thundering on the stairs. I renewed my advance and he fled. Finally with my group and the rightful owner of the house, we entered and took possession.

The Court bearer then made his appearance. Only after telephoning, did the police force arrive to help us. The culprits were loaded into the police van and taken for interrogation and safe custody. The incident was reported in the local newspaper the next day, with witnesses commenting on the "miracle" of my withstanding the barrage of soda bottles and stones!

Divine Healing:
The Dolphin experience of Matsyendranath

It was the 27th of July 1996. I was in Puna, on the big island of Hawaii. I rose early with the dawn to meet the Sun, rising majestically from the Pacific, as the massive red globe threw the Hawaiian skies into a splendid spectrum of colors. So ineffable was the ocean air, so rich and pristine, that all this left me lost inside myself. I sat for meditation on the lava cliff of our cottage overlooking the vast violet waters with the black Kahena Beach to my far left. This was heaven on earth.

Soon I became absorbed in *dhyana* and was oblivious to my surroundings. The occasional ocean waves thundered the very cliff I sat on and sprayed me even at a height of twenty feet. As I moved deeper into my Self, all this became a part of me. I felt calm, undisturbed and a deep gratitude to nature and its bounties arose in me. I had never ever felt the awesome Pacific, not so "pacific" that day, so intimately before. And there arose before me out of the ocean, the splendid form of the half-fish, half-man. This was the "Dolphin King" Matsyendranath, with his feet submerged in the ocean and his body soaring into the skies. I was overwhelmed with joy but could not understand the meaning of the vision. It became clear to me after I finished with this experience.

Then I heard one of my disciples call out, "They are here, the dolphins!" The house we were staying in had formerly belonged to her and she knew their ways and time. It's a rare thing to swim with dolphins in captivity, but it's totally out of this world to swim in the wild ocean with free dolphins. Knowing that this was not an opportunity to lose, I got up and made towards the black beach, as a group of my students followed behind. I always have my swim trunks on and other gear with me, at seaside resorts.

Usually the dolphins come quite close to shore and call out to the people to come play with them, but we went before that, and saw them at a distance spinning and jumping and diving as they glistened in the morning sunlight. As we swam out, we were cautious to go slowly and conserve our stamina for we had no idea how long it would take in this romance with the dolphins.

Being buffeted by the waves, up and down and sideways, we felt like paper boats. The waves were big yet friendly and the salinity of the ocean kept us easily afloat. Then as I dipped into the valley of a wave I couldn't see anything. The next swell of the wave raised me up and I saw the dolphins gracefully "dolphining" towards me. Before I could prepare myself to stroke them, they whizzed past me under the water with torpedo-like speed. The dolphins swim above the ocean in a wave-like motion, and under water they may adopt the same style, or shoot out like a torpedo. They are the smallest species of whales and can attain speeds of up to fifty kilometers an hour.

Like the dolphins, we also swam in pods for we were in the "great blue", the Pacific Ocean. We then spread out for there were five other dolphin lovers swimming with the dolphins. They were well equipped with their gear, flippers, snorkels and goggles. They had goggles and flippers - everything but no swim trunks, which in deep ocean waters didn't matter anyway. We on the other hand had only swimwear and none of the essential swim stuff, so our movements were slow and our vision under water was blurred. Our well-equipped natural naked guys were simultaneously able to breathe and look underwater to trace the hide-and-seek movements of the dolphins; so we took our queue from them.

However, even the slow movements of the dolphins were too fast for all of us, including those with fins. I was getting tired so I stretched out and lay afloat on the "ocean bed," with the swell and valley of the waves giving my body and bones a great massage. In the meanwhile, the news spread by word of mouth, or "coconut telegraph", that the new guru who had come, had gone into deep water with the dolphins. They showed concern that I should come back before the ocean got rough, as they had no idea how well I could swim and so some simple local folks prayed for my safety.

Very few people on the Big Island had phones. Even electricity had been discouraged by the locals. They even disapproved of geo-thermal power due to the toxins produced thereby. Only solar light lanterns seemed to work in the remote part of the big island they called Hawaii. They are careful not to corrupt nature in Hawaii. "This is the last frontier," they said, "let's keep the nature pristine here."

Suddenly a thought struck me as I lay afloat on the ocean bed, "Suppose I called out to them in a high pitch sound, would these highly developed playmates heed the call and come? Would they come if encased in my call was the emotion for help or distress?" So I tried the high pitched call in vowels such as *Eeee*, *Oooo* and *Ahhhh* but nothing happened. The dolphins didn't come. Perhaps I had gotten the song wrong, or was out of tune, I suppose. No matter how far they are, within moments the dolphins can come by you and in a trice they are gone. There were twenty to thirty dolphins that I saw swimming in unison and in a pod. The closest they came to me was about twenty feet, usually about fifteen to twenty feet away, but they surrounded us and flipped and played and sang.

Although this was already an experience of a lifetime, I wanted to touch a dolphin. The contact was of prime importance, but how could this happen? The ocean was swelling to roughness a bit as the waves crashed against the far away rocky shore. Then all of a sudden, as I lay afloat, a salty wave gushed up my nostrils, all the water up my nose. "Good for the sinus," I consoled myself and began to swim towards the dolphins. They were giving us the swim of our lives.

Then I decided to stop swimming. I held my breath, put my head underwater, and shut my mouth. Using my throat, I let out a high pitched sound of *Eeeeee*. I could barely raise my head up from the water and the whole school of dolphins swam under me, unbelievably close. How close I cannot say. I thought this was a fluke and that was that! I gave a few other underwater calls but to no avail. Although this was a trial and error experiment, I was aware that should I hit the correct pitch and frequency of sound, the dolphins would respond. Nature had made their receptive sound system to perfection.

Blissfully ignorant of the sonar communications system between them, I left it to the dolphins. I was having a bit of an aching spine and a pinched nerve was affecting my right leg. It was sciatica. They say that dolphins are sensitive to even body pain vibes. This time I inhaled deeply, shut my mouth and lips tight and with full force through my throat, let out the high pitched *Eeeeee* sound and continued long. The emotion infused in the sound was of happiness and help. I knew this was crazy and may not be in keeping with current scientific theory. But then again, how much does science know and how much does nature? She knows better. After all I bet you the first scientists who experimented must have tried some crazy things like this.

After I gave the call I rested and then I felt an exchange happening in a portion of my emotion. My devotion was being drawn out of me and simultaneously I was being replenished with a physical energy, an animal magnetism. No sooner had this happened, as I was treading water, I saw him come underwater, a solitary dolphin. He first steadied himself, studied me and then with accurate velocity, he grazed the right side of my pelvic bone from the front. Something in my lumber spine made a noise while my hands touched the smooth rubbery skin as he flowed by me. The rest of the group of dolphins swam underneath. When I tried to go after them, I realized how slow and cumbersome a mammal man is. I was a competitive swimmer in school, but this school of dolphins was just too fast for me to handle. But they often swim slowly for man and then what an experience to have with the free dolphins of the violet Pacific.

When I swam at Oahu, another island of Hawaii, the shallow waters were turquoise and crystal. Then, as we entered deeper waters it became blue and in very deep waters, it became violet. Such were the golden beaches of Lani Kai and Wahameha, with their forty-foot waves, which I was awed to see, during the stormy season. However, in the big Isle Hawaii, the waters from blue became violet very soon, indicating their great depth and charisma. Here the one hundred foot waves could be seen on stormy occasions and the proper season.

There is an age-old Hawaiian saying, "When the dolphins come out to play, the sharks never stay." The dolphins have the largest brain mass compared to all mammals in proportion to their size and can be compared to that of a human. What potential such a brain holds is still under research. But these aquatic friends show remarkable learning skills and a great friendship towards the human species. They have a surprisingly well developed neo-cortex, but how they use it is yet to be known by man who has not yet learned to fully use his own.

The ocean and the sky inspired me and I drank of God through nature. As I stepped on to the black beach of Kahena, lo and behold, my sciatica had been cured. Now I knew who had visited and cured me in the form of the big dolphin. He removed the sciatica of my leg so I could meditate unhindered by pain. The vision of Matsyendranath became clear reality to me.

> *The Sunset shades of melting hue*
> *White maned waves roll home*
> *Violet Ocean heavenly vault*
> *Melt in the selfsame dome.*

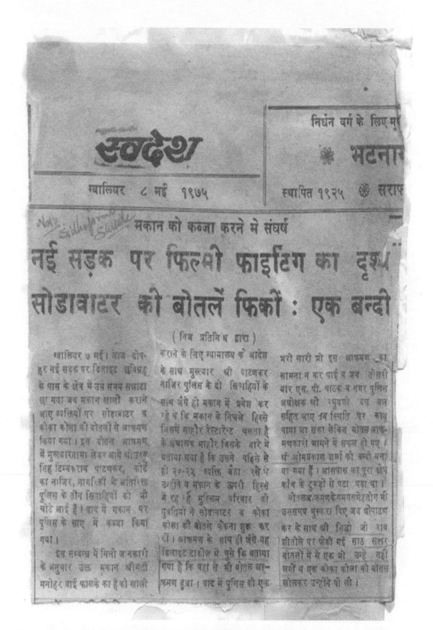

An account of Gurunath's incident where he created a shield of light (Surya Kavach) *to ward off stones and bottles thrown at him; given in the newspaper 'Swadesh' 8th May, 1975*

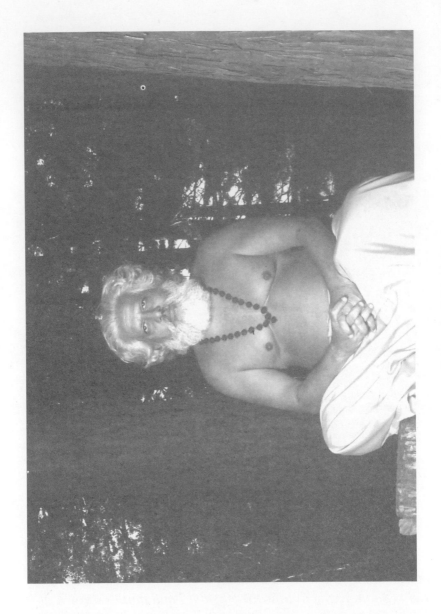

Yogiraj in Samadhi

CHAPTER 8

VANAPRASTHYA ASHRAM DAYS
The Forest Hermitage Of A Householder Yogi

Sitting in a shanty hut, I sipped a blessedly hot cup of tea. It was raining outside and the mist had covered the hilly ranges of Simhagadh Fort, near Pune. India has heavy rainfalls during the monsoon season and we were bang in the middle of it, being the month of August 1983. "What a beautiful place this Simhagadh (Lion Fort Valley) is for an *ashram*," I thought to myself. Just the day before a village friend called Bapu Paigude took my wife, Shivangini, and me to the valley called Sita Mai to see a proposed site for our *Hamsa Yoga ashram*.

The valley was called Sita Mai (the Mother Sita) because Rama, the ancient *avatar* savior of humanity, and his wife Sita tarried there for some days on their long journey from southern to northern India. So we decided to purchase this beautiful plot of land to build the *ashram*. We first got the water locations there by machine and by men who were waterfinders. When they told us that the area had water, we purchased the land in the Sita Mai valley near the Lion Fort Simhagadh.

There is a legend that the great *Rishi* called Kaundanya meditated there and hallowed the surroundings. The *ashram* site sits in a broad valley surrounded by hills on three sides. As one goes deeper towards the southeastern hills, after a good two kilometers, one comes upon a small water reservoir, near which is a *Shiva Linga* and a square box like stone with some difficult-to-identify stone sculptures. In the Sita Mai valley behind the *Shiva Linga*, there is a roughly-built waterhole for animals to come and quench their thirst.

Amidst the jungle terrain, two seasonal streams flow from the south to the north and from the east to the north-west of the *ashram*. The *ashram* was bought in 1983 and work began slowly as there were no funds to build it.

Shivangini put her heart and soul into building the first kitchen and pump house, with the help of some disciples. She built the kitchen with her own hands and the help of some local village masons. It was not an easy job and they wanted more money for the work. They exploited the situation because the work was in a forest area and no other labor was available. More often than not, we gave in to their demands.

Once, while building the underground septic tank of a bio-gas toilet, the chief mason suddenly decided to take further advantage of us, saying that he could not proceed with building the septic tank because there was no labor. So there I was, in the middle of this forest land with a few of my disciples who had come to visit. I told them to rise to the occasion since the bio-gas system had to be built before the rains. "Okay boys", I said, "take off your shirts and jump into the fray." To the utter consternation of the mason, we began digging the hole with our shovels and carrying bricks to the construction spot. The mason's plot to demand more money by obstructing our work was foiled. After a week of hard work by all of us *ashramites,* the bio-gas and toilet were completed.

There was and is no more a faithful a companion than Shivangini. The students affectionately call her "*Aie*," meaning, "loving mother," and they respect her as the *Gurumata* (Guru Mother) of the *ashram*. Night and day she worked and toiled to develop the *ashram* and bring it to what it is today. Throughout the summer heat she would not only supervise the *ashram* work, but participate in its development from planting the mango orchard with me, to the construction of the houses. Whether it was summer or winter, day or night, she was always on top of the job.

Once I went out at 1 o'clock in the morning and she was sleeping outside with our two boys, Shivraj and Rudrasen. They were sleeping like logs after their hike to Fort Simhagad. Shivraj was then about twelve years old and Rudrasen was ten. Where she slept with the boys was an open shed with no protection. I had a strange feeling that a panther was lurking nearby in the forest, but I was unsure of its presence. However, Shivangani got up in the middle of the winter night and made hot tomato soup with sippets. This was like a wonderful dream—she has always been so resourceful.

I got up at the crack of dawn, but Shivraj was already awake, and sure enough he showed me the leopard's pug marks. He was fond of tracking animals in the jungle and good at it too. The boys spent time with me in the forest *ashram* and were used to the jungle ways and adaptive life. The spotted beast had been lurking in the dark but did not attack any of my family members. They all had the habit of saying the protective *Gayatri mantra* before sleeping, as Shivangani had taught them. The smaller leopard species (pantherets), do not usually bother to attack humans as we are too big. Their main prey is the deer and the village dogs. But when a man is asleep, who can say?

Some of the spiritual experiences of the goddess Kali and the divine Nath beings that we had at the *ashram* are clearly etched in my memory. I shall relate a few. One night as we camped in the shanty pump house of the *ashram*, Shivangani was sleeping with a black cow near her cot. I kept night watch in the forest to prevent any stray hyenas and leopards from preying on our little black cow. As the night wore on, I was just nodding off when I heard a rustling in the bushes. In a moment I sat bolt upright and alert. But then I relaxed, reminding myself that the feline species were too stealthy to make any noise.

Just then a deer ran out of the thicket into the moonlight and made good its way across an open patch. It ran towards the deeper forest down south.

Later in the night, a whirlwind occurred in the *ashram*. In my twilight state, I heard the voices of many young ladies. Then I saw a strange vision. The goddess Kali came in all her finery with her divine *yoginis*. They began to dance the *Phugdi*, where two girls hold hands and spin round and round, going faster and faster until one gives up. I then fell off to sleep thinking that was just my dream, but when I got up the next morning, Shivangani related the same vision to me. I felt deeply grateful to the goddess Kali for blessing our *ashram*.

On the hill to the west there is a very small Kali place where the villagers go to worship. On the eastern hill I built the Shiva Temple. The *ashram* is a balanced activity of Yin and Yang, Shiva and Shakti. It would be no exaggeration to say that if it had not been for Shivangani's courage and determination, I alone would not have been able to develop the *ashram* to the stage at which it is today. The Lord in his grace has given me a wonderful partner. I am truly grateful for His grace, and my wife's devotion towards me, the *Hamsas* and the *ashram*.

The *ashram* flowered spiritually as we meditated and laughed and infused it with the dedication of *Hamsa* disciples and fervent devotions of our *bhajans* and chanting around the *dhuni* (the sacred night fires). This is now the *Tapo Bhumi*, the place of spiritual progress, kindled by intense meditation and joy. My writings have emerged in these sylvan surroundings. I wrote my poems the "Mystic Wine," "Cup of Tea," "Mind Transformation," and many a wondrous works were accomplished here.

So the Mother Center, the *Siddhanath Forrest Ashram*, imparts the Yoga of timeless evolution to all sincere seekers the world over during the New Life Awakening camps. Fostering among the peoples of the earth a realization that humanity is one's uniting religion, breath one's uniting prayer and consciousness one's uniting God. Let us accept our humanity for what it is and do what we must do to serve humanity as our larger Self.

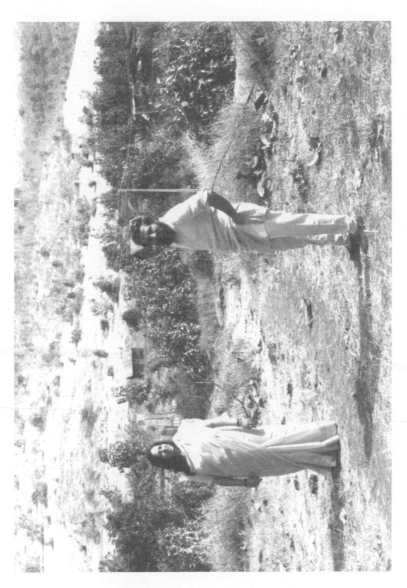

Yogiraj and Shivangini examining the land for the Ashram

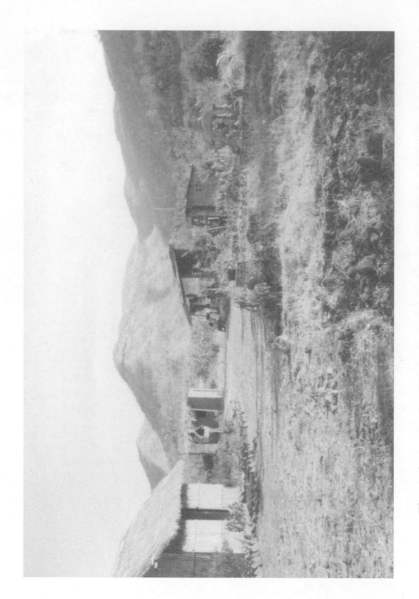

The Ashram in the 80's: rustic lifestyle conducive to meditation

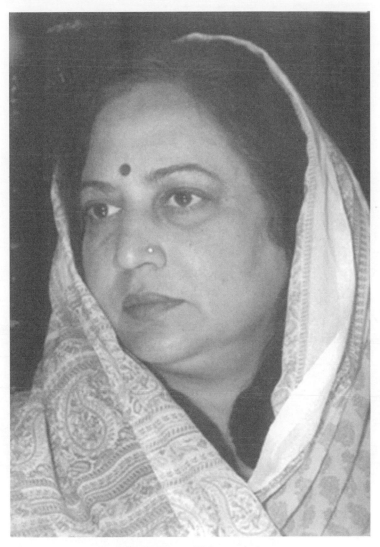

Gurumata Shivangini

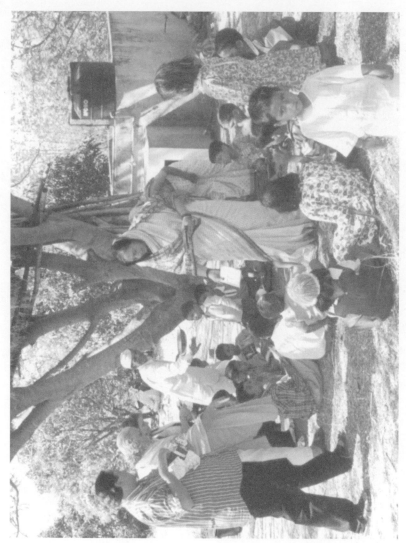

Yogiraj and Shivangini feeding the poor children

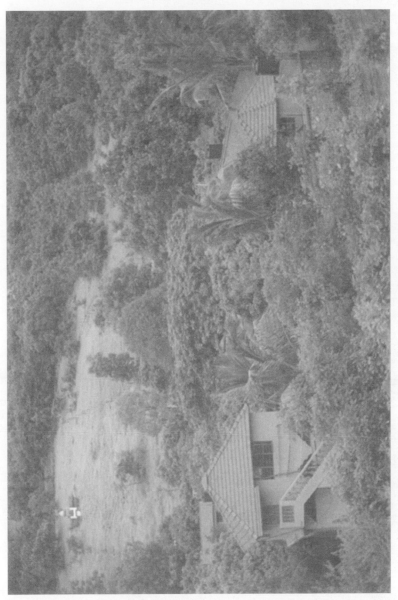

Panoramic view of the Siddhanath Forest Ashram in 2002

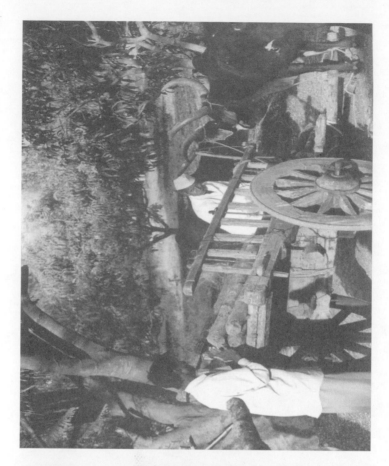

Villagers help with Ashram work

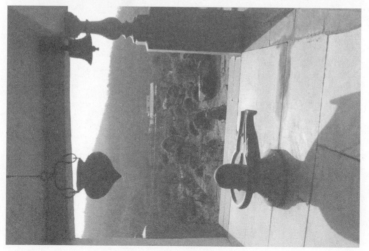

Shiva Temple in the Ashram

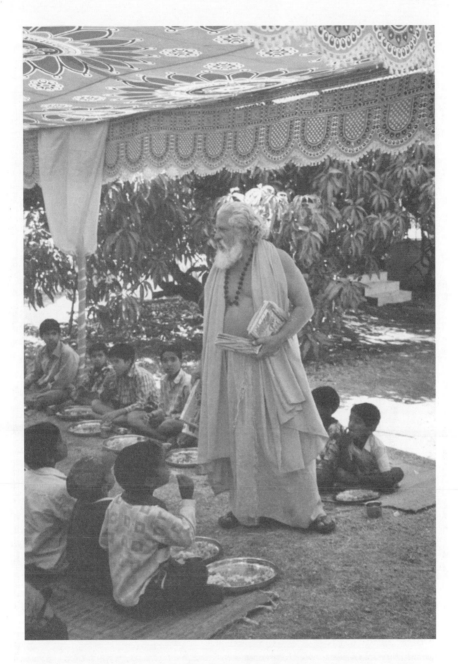

Yogiraj distributing books during the feeding of needy chidren

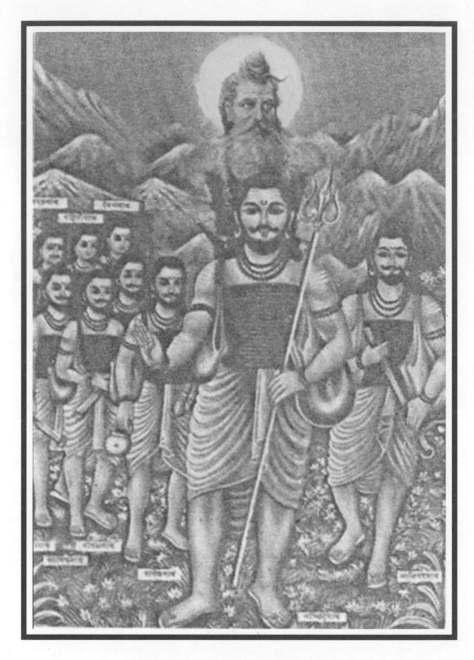

Originated from Adi Nath Shiva
The Nine Immortal Nath Yogis The Sages of the Fire Mist

CHAPTER 9

THE NINE NATHS OF IMMORTAL SPLENDOR

They are "the Ancient of Days," composed of the divine essence of the "Being About Whom Naught May Be Said." These immortal Divinities are ever watchful over the welfare and evolution of the destinies of nations and their humanities. Since they are *aja* (unborn) they can never die although their essences do incarnate for the salvation and evolution of humanity. I have detailed below an order of the celestial hierarchy of the heavenly host.

Lord Shiva

Parvati   *Alakh (Kartik)*

Maha-Maya   *Vishnu*

Chandrasoma   *Brahma*

Adi-Shesha   *Ganesh*

The Celestial hierarchy manifests as the corresponding Nine *Naths* below:

Babaji-Gorakshanath

Udai Nath   *Kartikeya*

Matsyendranath   *Rama(Shelnath)*

Chowrangnath   *Satyanath*

Achalachambunath   *Kanthadnath*

The Nine *Naths* are followers of Adinath Shiva and the Nath lineage represents one of the oldest yogic order ascetics whose origins are lost in the night of history. As I have mentioned, these *Nath Siddhas* are living in many secluded parts of India, mainly in the Himalayas. They guide the eighty-four *Siddhas* who form the Guardian Wall of

Humanity. These great *Naths* in everlasting meditation are infused in the Himalayan ranges, including the highest mountain called Gauri Shankar, which later a certain Mr. Everest named after himself.

Although the Nine Naths are Immortal, for the inspiration of humanity and for future generations to come, there are Nine sacred shrines (*samadhis*) in the Himalayas associated with the Nath tradition. They are Amarnath, Kedarnath, Badrinath, Pashu-Patinath, Kailashnath, Tunganath, Rudranath, Vishwanath (Kashi), and Jaggannath.

It is interesting to note that all of the Nine Naths have evolved beyond the sixth level of consciousness, called *Avadhoots*. Some of them, with tremendous yoga and *tapa*, have evolved to the *avasta* (state) of an Avatar Nath Yogi, beyond the seventh level of universal consciousness. Their consciousness is of such an advanced state that it is extremely difficult to comprehend their spiritual stature. A comprehensive description of these levels of consciousness is given in the chapter called "The Way of the White Swan".

Nath Yogis have also gone on to the eighth level of divine consciousness. They are known as *Rishis*, the custodians of our human evolution. These Sages of the Fire Mist are great beyond man's reckoning. Gautama Buddha, the fully enlightened, ascended to this eighth level. Lord Krishna, as Narayana, descended from it to be amongst mortals and hence was a *Purna Avatar*, the descent of Divinity in flesh. In the case of Matsyendranath and Jalandaranath, they ascended to achieve the state that Buddha had already attained and Krishna already was.

Still higher there is a great mystery and sacrifice involved in the ninth level of Divine Awareness. Such cosmic *avataric* descents are Self-taken and are one of a kind in human history, that is, each would be unique. These levels of spiritual consciousness are way beyond the understanding of human beings or *devas* (gods). The stupendous magnitude of their work is incomprehensible.

I have not written about all the primeval Nine Naths mentioned above. Instead I have given accounts of later Nath Yogis, with some of whom I've had personal experiences.

Adinath (Lord Shiva)

This means "the First Lord" who is Shiva himself, the unborn undying deathless "Lord of Liberating Yoga." He is the Eternal Now as Adinath, whose Self-taken work for the world cycle is to reabsorb an erring humanity into its original state of consciousness, by awakening them to and teaching them the Yoga of Self-Realization. Both the *Kaula* tradition of Matsyendranath and the Nath tradition of Gorakshanath acknowledge Him as their primal Lord and Master. Identified with Lord Shiva, he is held to be the original giver of divine *yogic* wisdom in a long line of masters and teachers of the *Yogachara* schools. The title Adi Nath is also given to Rishub Nath, the first of the twenty-four enlightened teachers called the "bridge builders" (*tirthankars*) of the Jain tradition, which is an integral part of the social and spiritual order of India.

Adinath was the primal Yogi and a direct manifestation of Shiva and it is from him that the yogis trace their lineage. He came much before the time of Minanath and is lost in the hoary antiquity of the misty past. His positive *shakti* energies are Umanath, Udainath, Parvatinath, Jagad Amba, Gauri and Bhavani. Some of His dark fiercer *shakti* energies are personified in Durga, Shyama, Chandi, Bhairavi, Chinna-masta and Kalinath. To balance the world, speed up evolution of souls and to accomplish what needs to be done, he may exercise any of his divine consort's *shakti* energies. To try and comprehend more would be futile in words. It would be more fruitful if we practice the ways to enlightenment and realize our true Selves.

Udainath (Parvati)

She is the manifestation of Parvati, the consort of Adinath Shiva. Udainath heralds the dawn of the age and time of spirituality. At one end, she helps the practitioner of yoga burn the seeds of all past negative *karma*s. On the other end, she supplies the light of inspiration to progress along the yogic path. She also plays the role of world mother and all throughout the passage of time she was the semi-divine Goddesss Renuka (the mother of Parashuram), Kaushalya (the mother of Ramchandra), Devaki (the mother of Krsna), Maya (the mother of Buddha) and Mary (the mother of Christ).

There are two aspects to her nature, one bright part, the other dark. In Shakti, the two aspects of Shiva are manifest. In her milder personification she is known as Uma, Gauri, Parvati, Jagadamba and Bhavani. In her dark and fierce character she is Durga, Shyama, Chandi Kali, Bhairavi.

Uma is the gracious consort of Adinath Shiva and the daughter of Prajapati Daksha. She, out of total love for Shiva, assumed a body so that she could be united with him in due form. This happening is related in the account of the sacrifice of Daksha as to how Shiva was insulted by not being invited to the sacrifice and later being ridiculed. This led to the violation and mortification of Uma, who then became Sati, sacrificed for the sake of her Lord. Then Shiva, grief-stricken, carried her over his shoulders telling Vishnu to dismember her. As he walked along, various parts of her sacred body fell at various sites, which now make the fifty-two holy *Shakti Pithas* (sacred places of worship).

After this she was reborn in the family of the sage Himavat and is thus called Parvati (daughter of the Himalayan Mountains). Shiva and Parvati are described as living together on the sacred Kailash Mountain. They are ever immersed in the *samadhi* of love, at times engaged in deep philosophical discourse to show the path of salvation to humanity lost in the theories of a material world. From these discourses many a treatise on Yoga and Tantra have been gifted to the world. These priceless treasures are their blessings to humanity and have been the cause of the liberation and bliss for countless yogis, saints, and common souls the world over. Parvati, of a darker complexion spiritually sought a more perfect attunement with her Lord in *samadhi* to match and totally merge into her Lord's being and becoming. So she took to severe penance (*tapasya*), the result of which was that she was transformed in body, mind, and spirit to a light golden color, assuming the form and name of Gauri (fair). She is also called Jagad Amba, the "fathomless deep of the universe."

When we go on to the more formidable aspects of Shakti, let us not for a moment forget, as many western writers do, the spirit of love and of the evolutionary push for the souls' salvation, which the Divine Mother has for us in her heart. Durga "the Unconquerable" is Adinath Shiva's consort in the aspect of warrior. She derives her name from the demon she slew. She is often depicted with eight arms (*Asta Bhuja*) during the festival of the nine nights of prayers (*Navaratri*).

Then we have the four-armed Kali with sword and a garland of heads around her neck, her red tongue protruding, thirsty for the blood of the demonical forces and demons. She is ever ready to destroy their outer body garments in her fierce compassion to liberate their souls to a higher form of life and awareness. The darker the negativity and evil on this earth, the fiercer and more aggressive her form becomes to overcome the evil and create a balance of the *gunas*. She is then Kala Bhairavi and Chinnamastu, where she cuts off her head and the triple sprouts of blood are drunk by her assistant *yoginis* and her own severed head. The Mother will go to the farthest extremes to liberate her children's souls from ignorance and hell damnation. She shows here that sacrifice is the ultimate solution to spiritual evolution and the attainment of *Brahma Nirvana*.

Matsyendranath

There is a legend of the Naths that, one day as the great Yogi sat fishing in his boat in the Bay of Bengal, he hooked a huge fish that pulled so hard on his fishing line that his boat capsized and the whale swallowed him whole. This is similar to the Biblical story of Jonah in the stomach of a whale. Now Matsyendranath was protected by his good *karma*. At that time, the Lord Shiva had created a beautiful setting under the ocean. He was expounding to his spouse, Parvati, the sacred doctrine of Yoga and *Tantra*, which he had never given to anyone else. The large fish happened to go to this very site.

So it came to pass that the Nath was able to hear the secret discourse which Shiva gave to Parvati, without being noticed. After some time Parvati fell asleep, and when Shiva asked, "Are you listening?" A prompt "Yes!" came from the belly of the fish. Using his *Shiva Netra* (third-eye), Shiva gazed into the belly of the fish where he saw Mina Nath (another of Matsyendranath's many names). He was overjoyed at the discovery and said, "Now I know who my real disciple is." Turning to his sleepy spouse He said, "I will now first initiate Matsyendranath," who gratefully took the initiation and then for the next twelve years, all the while remaining in the belly of the fish, dedicated himself to the *Tantra Yogic* practices given to him by the Lord Shiva himself. At the end of the twelve years another fisherman caught the monster and, upon opening it, Matsyendranath appeared as a fully realized Master.

Matsyendranath is responsible for the transmigration of all evolving souls. In his hands are the keys to the gates of salvation (*moksha*). He gives liberation to the deserving and bondage to fools. He is the immortal Master of *Hatha* and *Tantra Yoga*. His *deva* form is called Avalokiteshwara, which means "The Lord Who Looks Down from On High". In Tibet he is the Bodhisattva Avalokiteshwara who gave to humanity the liberating mantra "*Om mani padme hum*". In Nepal he is venerated as the guardian deity of Kathmandu in the form of Shveta Matsyendra (White Fish Lord). In India he is the

Nath, Matsyendra celebrated in song and legend as the savior and spiritual redeemer of all the Nath Yogis. In his *Tantra Aloka*, the great Abhinav Gupta salutes Matsyendranath as his *Guru*. The book called *Kaulu-Jnana-Nirnaya*, meaning "ascertainment of *Kaula* Knowledge," was authored by Matsyendranath around the tenth century and is one of the oldest available sources of information about *Kaulism*.

According to a legendary account in this book, he is said to have recovered the canon of the *Kaulas* called *Kulagama* from a large fish that had swallowed it. He is specifically associated with the *Kaula* sect of the *Siddha* movement, within which he founded the *Yogini-Kaula* branch. This *tantric* sect derives its name from the word "*Kula*," which is the ultimate reality in its dynamic feminine aspect called *Kundalini Shakti*. The word *Kula* has various meanings. One meaning is "flock" or "multitude," but more significantly it means "family of respect". It is thus called the *Kula Kundalini* because it is both the source of many multi universes as well as the final home and security for *yogis* who awaken and abide in her secrets. The Lord Shiva in Tantrism is called *Akula*, that which transcends all dualities and differences. Therefore the concept of *Kaula* stands for the *avasta* (state) of enlightenment gained through the union of Shiva and Shakti. *Kaula* also refers to a practitioner of this path.

Shiva-Goraksha-Babaji

There is a great mystery and a sacrifice associated with the ninth level of Divine awareness which is Self-born. This is the state of *Brahma Nirvana* from which the ineffable Shiva-Goraksha-Babaji descends. He comes to redeem humanity yet maintains his state. How this is possible is known only to him.

He is the protector of the cattle (*gow-raksha*). He symbolizes cow ash, the *vibhuti* of the *dhunis* (sacred fires) of all Nath Yogis. He is the good shepherd who guides the sheep from the dangerous mountains to the safety of green pastures. He is the Lord of animals (*Pashupati*) who transforms our animal passions into the love for God. Such is our savior, the Yogi Messiah of humanity.

He is the collective consciousness of the seven primordial Sages of the Fire Mist born at the beginning of time. He is the total light of the highest Elohim and yet in his unfathomable compassion, has left behind a finite portion of his infinite consciousness to evolve humanity into the likeness of Divinity. This finite and immortal portion of his Divinity manifests among the haunts of men from time to time as the need arises. Throughout eternity this Eternal Now watches over the evolution of humanity till the time it is liberated. Truly, he is called "the Great Sacrifice," the Visible Invisible Savior of Mankind.

Babaji is ever the same. He was never born and therefore can never die. They call him *Aja* (the unborn). But from time to time this compassionate Lord of irradiant splendor does manifest for humanity. Pulling the veil of *maya* by his own will, He takes a form of lightless light to incarnate among mortal beings. He guards, guides, and enlightens their consciousness as per their evolutionary blueprint. His deathless body of lightless light may take any form through which he can express and reveal Himself to the faithful from age to age.

Shiva himself took the form of Shiva Goraksha Babaji then of Rudra of the Ancient of days. He then manifested in 6000BCE as Kal Agninath. Subsequently, he came in 500BCE in the holy city of Kashi as Dakshinmurti, during which he initiated himself. In the year 70BCE he manifested himself as Gorakshanath, at the time of King Shalivahan and Chowrangeenath. Still later, the ever-present Babaji Goraksha journeyed north to Nepal where he conquered the Nagas and was called Nagaraja (not to be confused with the hypothetical Nagraj of South India). The Nagas are a certain type of yogi practitioners who assumed the form of *nagas* (cobras). They hold the mystic knowledge of *Kundalini* awakening. In the same ever-present immortal body he later appeared as Shiva-Goraksha-Babaji in the 9th century CE. This was during the time of Guganath whom He empowered to have complete mastery over the Nagas and ultimately be worshipped as a Naga god himself.

Babaji Gorakshanath is himself shown in the supreme *samadhi* sitting as Nagaraj upon a yogic throne under which are the Nine Nagas: Vasuki, Ananta, Takshaka, Varuna, Padmaka, Sankhpala, Kulika, Mahapadma, and Karkotaka. Then the Lord of *karma* and destiny, Shiva-Goraksha-Nagaraj, sat upon his throne to withhold the rain for twelve years and create a drought to give the people of Nepal their *karmic* retribution, thereby evolving their souls. The snakes that were subdued to form his *asana* throne were: Varuna (white in color and wearing a sevenfold jeweled "*naga*-hood"), Ananta (carrying a jewel in a lotus in his hands and taking his position in the center of a dark blue hue in the east), Padmaka (the color of a lotus stalk with five hoods in the south), Takshaka (the nine-hooded and saffron colored in the west), Vasuki (the seven-headed green taking his position in the north), Shankha pala (yellowish in the south-west), Kulika (the white with thirty heads in the northwest), Karkotaka (the half-human with the snake tail of a blue color in the southeast), and Mahapadma (golden-colored in the northeast). When the souls of Nepal had been purged of their sins, Matsyendranath appeared in Nepal, then Gorakshanath got up to greet him, and the Nagas were released and there was copious rainfall.

In another story it so happened that the great Matsyendranath journeyed to the Himalayas and there carried out intense tapa and meditation. Then Adinath, Lord Shiva was pleased and appeared to the Nath, to ask him what he needed. The great yogi asked Shiva to give him a disciple greater and more perfect than himself. The Lord answered and said, "You are already perfect and have attained to the final enlightenment." But Matsyendranath insisted, so Lord Shiva said that he would himself manifest as his disciple. Then, from the heart of Shiva (who is the Eternal Shiva-Goraksha-Babaji) burst forth an irradiant flame of splendor and Shiva-Goraksha-Babaji was manifest in the causal realm and later by the power of *Kriya Shakti*, he involuted to pull around himself a vesture composed of sub-atomic particles of light, creating an *avataric* body to manifest on the terrestrial plane.

Then the Lord of compassion Shiva-Goraksha-Babaji initiated his mission to cleanse and free the earth and its people from the mire of materialism and ignorance that cover their souls, to give to them the radiant love and nectar of the Divine through *Kriya Yoga* meditation.

Babaji's Yoga and *Kriya Yoga* teachings are found in his sacred book called *Goraksha Paddhati*, which was later compiled by a certain Svatmarama Yogi into the famous *Hatha Yoga Pradipika* in the Middle Ages. In more recent times, Babaji gave to Yogavatar Lahiri Mahasaya, the *Kriya Yoga* teachings adapted to suit the evolution of today's peoples.

Gorakshanath had assumed legendary fame during his manifestation in the Middle Ages. Many stories of other saints competing with the Nath are of a sectarian prejudice and show a total disregard for the dates and era in which Goraksha existed historically. It came to be established that no saint or yogi was considered to be of any worth or importance unless and until he had defeated the legendary Gorakshanath in a contest of yogic powers or in a philosophical debate. And so the disciples of those respective saints or yogis saw to it that they defeated the Nath even if a false story had to be concocted and even if Gorakshanath predated those later saints by a good two to three hundred years. Everything was disregarded by these fanatic followers in their fervor, to acclaim their respective Guru Masters as the "bestest" and "mostest," if I may use such terms. There are stories of Allam Prabhu, Kabir, and Nanak in this context, saints who came much later than Gorakshanath. Of course, those great beings had no hand in the distorted literature written in their praise, a false praise they were certainly not in need of. Svatmarama Yogi names Allam Prabhu as one of the disciples of Goraksha. There seemed to be a rift between disciples with interpolations in their scriptures that do not match the dates of the original documents nor the claims they make. Gorakshanath was beyond doubt the Supreme Master of both Allam Prabhu and Naga Arjun.

My reason for elaborating on the manifestation of Shiva-Goraksha-Babaji during the Middle Ages is because he made known the great sacrifice to liberate all sentient and insentient beings for the whole world cycle during that time and therefore is called *Mahabhinishkaran* or "Great Sacrifice". His notable appearances were:

- Shiva appears to Goddess Ambika as Shiva-Goraksha-Babaji while She was meditating at Gorakh Math in Girnar, showing that Babaji is Shiva himself.
- Kabir, the medieval saint, praises Shiva-Goraksha-Babaji and Gopichand. He is indebted to them for initiating him into the Knowledge of *Kundalini Kriya Yoga*, six *chakras*, *Shabda Yoga*, and *Omkar* meditation.
- The great Shiva-Goraksha-Babaji taught to Guru Nanak the *Surat Nam Yoga*, *Shabad* (*Shabda Yoga*) and *Omkar* meditation.
- Later, Guru Nanak's *Japji* prayer book makes it a point to mention Goraksha's name with Shiva, Parvati, *etc.* showing the high esteem in which he was held in Nanak's time, being worshipped with the Gods.
- Swatmarama Yogi records Allam Prabhu and Naga Arjun as disciples of Gorakshanath. Allam was born 150 years after the historically mentioned Gorakshanath.

Illustrative Parables

On Renunciation

Once a householder came to pay his respects to the Maha Yogi Goraksha with folded hands, he said, "Oh Respected One, your sacrifice is great, for you have given up the whole world for God." Goraksha replied with folded hands, "Oh Respected One your sacrifice is greater than mine for you have given up the infinite God for this finite world."

On Death

A practicing yogi full of rage at his failure to attain samadhi was on his way to die Goraksha was sitting calmly under a tree and asked, "Where are you going my son?" "To die!" replied the frustrated yogi. Goraksha said, "Then die if you must but make sure the dying is complete. If you cannot do it, come to me, I will teach you to die so completely that you will never die again and become deathless (*amar*). The *yogi* came back and attained to deathless *samadhi* under the loving eye of his guru, Shiva-Goraksha-Babaji.

King Guganath – The Chauhan (970CE-1000CE)

Born on the 8th day of Bhadon (Shravan Bhadrapad), he was the son of King Jewar and Queen Bacchal of the Agni Vamsha lineage of the Chauhan clan of Rajputs. By the grace and blessings of the Divine Guru Gorakshanath, at his birth a *naga* appeared and he was later worshipped as a *Naga* god. To this day, in my family temple at Gwalior, victims of snake and scorpion bites are cured. To this day, women desirous of good children pray and their prayers are granted.

I was born on the 10th of May, in 1944, by the blessings of Gorakshanath Babaji, through the grace and holy ash of my family Guru, Guganath. Babaji blessed me with his Presence and is till this moment ever guiding me in my service to humanity, giving through me the path of yogic meditation for the evolution of human consciousness. My whole life, during my Himalayan travels and my teachings in India and America, I am breathed through by Guganath and Gorakshanath's inspiration.

The temple my grandfather, the late Raja Shitole Deshmuk of Pune, built in Gwalior is dedicated to Guganath. The sanctum sanctorium (the holy of holies) is dedicated to his great Guru Gorakshanath. Even today, a *Guru Darbar* (royal court of the Guru) is held every Monday at Mahal Goan in Gwalior, in the state of Madhya Pradesh, and attended by my family. We are welcomed and honored by the beating of drums as we enter the temple marking the family status of a Raja (King). By tradition and the wish of King Guganath, our family is made to sit on the left outside of the inner sanctum of Shiva-Goraksha-Babaji. To the right side sits the officiating priest and directly in front of the Gorakshanath altar room a throne of flowers is laid for King Guga, the Chauhan.

After some time, the *Mahant* (head priest) of the temple, who is infused with the holy spirit of Guga, sits in front of the sanctum. Before the ceremony, a sacred fire, infused with the holy Spirit of Guganath, is lit by the priest to invoke and to honor the Maha Guru Shiva-Goraksha-Babaji. Camphor, clarified butter, incense, saffron and sandalwood are used to invoke the Presence of the Divine Goraksha. Petitions are made as the priest brushes the petitioner with a brush of peacock feathers (*morchal*).

The *Mahant* loses all body consciousness as he is inspired by the great Soul of Guga Nath who uses his body as an instrument to deal with the victims of snake and scorpion bites. The body with the spiritual entry (*avesh*) of great Guru Guga grants boons to the faithful. All wishes that are worthy of being granted are granted by the Chauhan Guganath. This is done in witness of the sacred fire of Gorakshanath. To barren women are granted children, to the sick their health, to snake-bitten people their cure, when their string bonds (*bandhas*) are cut in front of the Goraksha fire. To the *yogis* are granted their spiritual success and an everlasting love for God and Goraksha (Guru Maharaj*)*.

I had been witnessing the Monday *Guru Darbar* my whole life till I grew up and finally met both these legendary *Gurus*. They have graced my livingness and made it worth living for others, making me realize that in serving humanity, I serve my larger Self.

When *T*akshaka Naga, the chief of the King Vasuki Naga, asked Guga the Chauhan about his ancestry, Guga replied, "I am the grandson of King Amar. I come from the village Gard Darera in Bikaner. I am the son of King Jewar Chauhan. My mother is Queen Bacchal. My name Guga is given to me by my *Maha Guru* Gorakshanath. By the blessings of Gorakshanath will be my marriage to Princess Sharada of Assam." Indeed Goraksha materialized a grand marriage party with elephants, horses, men and jewelry to marry his disciple King Guga with unparalleled pomp and splendor.

His mother Bacchal, who had formerly left her King, went to her home in Fort Gazni, which was located in Kabul. So this would connect Guganath with the Rajputs reigning in Kabul before the *Mussalman* (Muslim) rule there. The Ratannath shrine also is near Kabul and so is the Khwaja Khizra shrine located in upper Sindh in Uderolal. This would also connect to the shrine of Kwaja Moin Uddin Chiste in Ajmer, both of whom were disciples of Shiva-Goraksha. There is a Gazni in Gujarat, which may have been the home of Queen Bacchal.

Raja Bhartrinath (1010CE-1126CE)

The last *Chandravat Raja* of the Parmars was Bhartrinath[*], the King of Ujjain. He abdicated the throne after the death of his queen Rani Pingala, and took the vow of sanyas, becoming a Goraknathi. His younger brother Vikramaditya (Chandragupta II) succeeded him to rule Ujjain from 1076-1126CE. It was Bhartrinath who directed Vikramaditya to renovate and rebuild the sacred city of Haridwar.

There is the famous story of how the King Bhartri, wanting to test his queen's love for him, sent a false message of his death to her. Although her *Asso Pat* plant (given to her by *Datta Guru*) revealed to her that the King was alive, she decided to prove her fidelity to him by dying on the funeral fire. The King, anxious about the result of his message, arrived at the palace only to see the funeral pyre. He wandered around the cremation site for days refusing to be comforted. Gorakshanath, who happened to pass by, asked the King the reason for his mourning and was told that it was due to the loss of his beloved queen. Thereupon Gorakshanath dropped and broke his begging bowl and began to sorrow and weep in imitation. The King, aghast, reminded Gorakshanath that his loss was neither so precious nor so irreparable as his—there never could be another queen such as Rani Pingala had been. Gorakshanath then sprinkled water over the ashes of the funeral pyre and showed him twenty-five queens exactly like Pingala. On sprinkling the water a second time, only Pingala remained. When she stood before the King alive, he refused to embrace her since, in his despair, he had renounced the world and he resolved to remain faithful to his sacred vow. More water was sprinkled by Gorakshanath and, casting a reproachful look at Bhartrinath, the queen disappeared.

---

[*] Referred to as *Barthahari* in chapter Six

The Queen *Pingala's* reproachful look certainly had in it the seeds for a *karmic* union in the next life. Both King Bhartri and Queen Pingala, although perfected beings, had to reincarnate in a future life. The great Shiva-Goraksha-Babaji could have liberated Bhartrinath to higher realms of *Nirvana*, but he chose to keep the seeds of desire in both their minds so that they could reincarnate on their *avataric* mission to teach to the world the divine science of *Kriya* and *Kundalini Yoga*. The two desires embedded in the mind of Bhartri were to make *karmic* amends to his wife by marrying her in the next life and to experience, even if for a short while, the life of royalty in a palace made of gold.

It is interesting to note that both these desires were fulfilled by Babaji to Lahiri Mahasaya who was first married to Kashi Moni and then came to the Himalayas where Goraksha-Babaji materialized for him a golden palace. Babaji had kept within them their desires for a purpose in a future life, to enable such a lofty *avataric* Soul to descend and complete its mission at the appropriate time.

My actually seeing Bhartrinath at Ujjain and my later vision of him at the Shipra river, where he transformed into Kabir and then into the smiling Lahiri Mahasaya corroborate the above fact. There is a good two to three hundred years gap between the incarnations of Bhartri, Kabir and Lahiri Mahasaya, all of whom had a mission to fulfill. My ancestral Raja Shitole family temple of Lord Rama is near the great Mahan Kaal Temple of Lord Shiva. Both Temples are in the vicinity where I had the experience of Lord Bhartrinath and Lahiri Mahasaya

There are two masterly works of literature written by the author Bhartrinath. The name of one of these books is the *Shrinagar Shatak* and the other work is *Vairagya Shatak*. The *Shrinagar Shatak* talks about the royal life, the ways of nuptial and decorative life-style of beauty, and *maya*. The *Vairagya Shatak* is a composition of dispassion and abandonment, the life and path of a yogi, the path of sacrifice and renunciation.

Kalagni Nath (6000BCE-reign of King Mahandatta)

This great *Nath yogi* is from the ancient of days as he lives on from age to age. No definite time frame is given for his work or mission. He predated the *Buddha* and his two Indian teachers, *Aradhya Kalam* and *Udraka Ramputra*. He in all probability taught them the great *Nath yogic* tradition of India, which was later passed on to *Gautama* the *Buddha*. The various names by which this mysterious being is mentioned are *Kalagni Nath, Kalaginath, Kalinath* and *Kalonos*.

Kalagni Nath, who belonged to the *Nav-Nath* (Nine Nath) tradition, appeared in *Varanasi* (Benares), India, around 600BCE. He initiated the *Siddha Bhoga Nath* of Benares into the Divine *Nath Yoga* as well as taught him the science of immortality called *Sanjeevani Vidya*, where the aging process of the body is arrested and the *yogi* can live for an indefinite period of time. This ancient *Nath* science of *Yoga* called *Sanjeevani Samadhi* (*Svaroop Samadhi*) was taken by *Bhoga Nath* from Benares to the south of India and came to be known as *Saroub Samadhi* in *Tamil*. In South India *Bhoga Nath* is popularly known as *Bogarnatha*. He further traveled to China where he was known as *Bo Yang* or *Lao-Tze*, and revolutionized China with his *yogic* teachings of body immortality and Tao Te Ching. He taught Golden Immortality and Yin Yang *Yoga*, where Yin, the *Kundalini* energy, rises, piercing the six *chakras*, and unites with Yang, her Lord *Shiva*, in *sahasrara*.

Kalagni Nath, a master of *Kaya Kalpa* and *Sanjeevani Samadhi* lived during the time of Alexander the Great when the conqueror entered the borders of India. His soldiers were exhausted after defeating the King *Porus*. Alexander's army was ready to beat a retreat when he happened to meet this great *yogi, Kalagni Nath*, whom the Greeks called *Kalanos*.

The great conqueror sent his soldiers to summon the *yogi* whom he found to be most enigmatic and intriguing. The soldiers said to

Kalagni, "The son of Zeus calleth Thee." The yogi replied, "Tell Alexander that there waiteth for him another son of Zeus and if he had need of me, he should come himself." Alexander came to meet Kalagni and offered him anything he wished for. The yogi smiled and asked him to step aside for he was blocking the sunlight, something Alexander could not give him. Alexander was humbled by this yogi. He owned nothing and yet made him feel so inadequate, that he requested Kalagni to accompany him to Greece. Several years later, the yogi lit his own funeral pyre in front of the Macedonian Army and entered the flames. As he went in, he told Alexander he would meet him in Macedonia. Then sitting in lotus posture he calmly let the flames consume what was to him his illusionary body.

Later on as Alexander lay dying on his bed in Macedonia, the Great Sage of the ancient of days kept his word and appeared by the bedside of the emperor. He told the monarch to instruct his servants to keep his empty hands out of his grave after he died. This was to teach the world a lesson that, be it the emperor of the world or be it an ordinary man, both come into the world with nothing and depart with nothing. Only Divine-realization is everlasting as Kalagni Nath proved to Alexander in life and in death with his own immortality and his Divinity.

Chowrangeenath (10BCE-103CE)

The Immortal *Naths*, although fully enlightened, spurned the final liberation of *Brahma Nirvana* to remain on earth for the instruction and guidance of humanity to Divinity. Amongst such saviors one of the foremost names is *Gyan Swaroop* (Divine form of Wisdom of Chowrangeenath).

Chowrangeenath, also called *Puran Bhagat,* was the son of King Shalivahan of the Rajput Parmars of Sialkot in the then Northern Punjab bordering Afghanistan. The King had two queens, the older of whom was Queen Archan, the Mother of Puran. The other queen, who was much younger, was barren. She made advances to Puran, which he refused, and so she brought false charges against him, which the King believed. Then cutting off Puran's hands and feet, he threw him into a well to die. This was the well in the village of Karol, five miles from Sialkot. It is now called Puranwala.

Gorakshanath happened to pass by to drink water and found the body in the well. Knowing Puran's innocence, He rescued the body from the well, brought it back to life and restored its limbs. *Puran* became a *Goraknathi* and followed the path of Yoga. He was given the name of Chowrangeenath. Such was his power and compassion that later he even granted his former betrayer, Queen Lunan, a boon. She bore a son named Rasalu, the legendary hero who conquered most of the cities in Afghanistan. Rasalu had a checkered life of romance, adventure and intrigue. His conquests in India and Afghanistan were due to the blessings of Gorakshanath whose ardent disciple he later became. He was the legendary hero conqueror and king whose name is mentioned with awe in Moslem history and documents.

It is interesting to note that it was during the reign of Emperor Kanishka of the Kushan Dynasty that these incidents and exploits occurred. The emperor himself was keen to combine the ancient Indian, the modern Greek and the Buddhist philosophies and revel in that knowledge. At that time, 10BCE-70CE, there happened to be, at Kashmir, the *Bodhisattva* Ishanath today called Jesus. Jesus, who had come to India to study Yoga, and Chowrangeenath, already a Great yogi, attended the great Buddhist council of Haran near Sri Nagar. There the collection of Buddha's work *Lalita Vistara* was formulated, which shows striking similarity with the New Testament.

An account of the meeting of King Shalivahan with Jesus is given in the ancient Indian text called the *Bhavishya Purana*. This is an historical account, which continues to be updated as historical events happen on earth. The *purana* means old book; it is the historical

171

account of a day of *Brahma* lasting 4,320,000,000 years. It is mentioned here that King *Shalivahan* met Jesus in Kashmir where the two exchanged views and *Shalivahan* later advised *Isha* (Jesus) to get married since he had finished his mission, which was announced in the year 54CE. The *Nath* Tradition of *Yoga*, by the time of Jesus' advent, was of hoary antiquity. It had a deep influence on Jesus' *yogic* and meditative practices. Tutored by his Guru Chetannath, Jesus went by the name of Ishanath.

Ishanath – Jesus (16BCE-104CE)

From my school days I was deeply intrigued by the life of Jesus and his missing years in the bible. So I set about spending a good deal of my time researching in books and documents for the missing years of the man Jesus and his connection to the immortal Christ and Christos. Besides the Dead Sea Scrolls, I feel that ancient documents found in a place called Nag Hammadi provide valuable details of Jesus' life.

It was during the time of the great Kushan dynasty and the rule of the benevolent King Kanishka I (78BCE-103CE), that Jesus came to India to learn the science of Yoga and immortality. In the mystical order of *Nath Yogis* (also called *Goraknathis*), there are the *sutras* known as *Nath Namavali*, which tell us of a saint called *Ishanath* who is said to have come from Nazareth to India at the age of fourteen. The name of his Indian teacher is mentioned as Chetannath, who taught Jesus the Yoga and its divine revelations. It is said that by his yogic powers he was able to survive his crucifixion on the cross and finally by these yogic powers (*siddhis*) of his *Guru*, Chetannath, he came once more to India. Here, he is said to have founded an *ashram* monastery amidst the foothills of the Himalayan Mountains.

The coming of Jesus was at the time when *Mahayana Buddhism* was popular and therefore he would have been influenced by those teachings of the Buddha too. Contrary to other orders and sects of Hinduism, the *Nath Yogis* do not recognize any caste system nor the supremacy of the high priests (*brahmins*). They look upon all people as equal - kings and carpenters, low and high, rich and poor are treated as children of God and are initiated into the *Nath* order. It is difficult to miss the attitude of Jesus towards the Gentiles, Samaritans, and the sinners when he sat down and ate with them. He was practicing the *Nath* way of life, equality to all human beings.

As it stands today, modern research shows in the life of Jesus a vacuum. In the gospels, he is missing abruptly from the age of thirteen till the age of thirty. This absence in the Bible is filled by his travels and stay in India, the spiritual dynamo of the world. There does not appear to be any historically reliable source or any information in the Bible during these seventeen years of his absence. Suddenly at the age of thirty, Jesus appears in the Bible to be baptized by John. Now during this period his travels and his stay have been authentically recorded in documents, scrolls and literature found in India.

A certain order of the *Nath Yogis* is characterized by their all encompassing compassion. Such yogis take on the suffering of all beings to redeem their sins and lead them to liberation. Those great yogis sacrifice nirva*na* for the redemption of the *karma* of mankind even if it means taking on themselves the suffering and guilt of humanity. All these characteristics are to be found in Jesus and his mission. The *Nath* sacrifice, the *Bodhisattva* philosophy of the Buddha, and Jesus' role of the sacrificial lamb all complement one another.

Lord Matsyendranath called Avalokiteshw*ara* (he who looks down in compassion), the Avatar of Narayana, has been portrayed in visual painting with marks of the stigmata on the surface of his hands and feet. Western scholars have recognized the stigmata of Jesus in the wheel signs and equate Matsyendranath, the Lord of Compassion, with Jesus, both of whom are *Bodhisattvas* as per the Buddhist philosophy. Avalokitesvara is the immortal (Christ) principle of Jesus the man as he lives immortal and is now merged in the Christos, also called eternal Narayana.

In the second chapter of the *Bhavishya Purana* (V/S 17-32) during the reign of Shalivahan, a clear account of the King's meeting with Jesus is given. This definitely goes to show that Shalivahan's son Chowrangeenath, Jesus (Ishanath), and his *Guru*, Chetannath, were all of the same period. Gorakshanath initiated Chowrangee and he, along with the other Naths, became *chiranjeev*, immortal *Naths*, the guardians of the Himalayan peaks and of humanity.

Fatima, the daughter of Muhammed the Prophet, had heard from him that the Prophet Jesus (*Yuz Asaf*) lived till the ripe old age of 120 after he recovered from his crucifixion. According to *yogic* tradition, this is called one human *kalpa* (*Kans-ul Ammal* Vol. II p. 34).

Though the mortal remains of Jesus lie buried in the Hazrat Issa Tomb in Kashmir, his Immortal spirit pervades the Badrinath area of the Himalayas, merged in his Christos (Narayana) who is to return to the world as the Kalki Avatara for the Hindus, Maitreya Buddha for the Buddhists, Imam Mahdi for the Muslims, and the second advent of Christ for the Christians. Which portion of the collective consciousness of God Narayana shall reincarnate, Jesus or another flame, is yet to be seen.

Jnannath – Lord of Wisdom (13th century CE)

The saint Jnaneswar was truly called the king of mystics in that he completed his famous book in his teens, the Jnaneshwari, a marvelous translation of the holy Bhagavad Gita of Lord Krishna. After having completed this work Jnannath (also Gyannath) took sanjeevan samadhi at Alandi, a small village near the town of Pune in India. When he went into his final samadhi, he was only eighteen years of age.

He was an adept in the *Nav-Nath* tradition of Yoga by which he achieved his *nirvikalpa samadhi* and *sanjeevan samadhi* states of final liberation. His spiritual lineage is from Gorakshanath-Babaji whose disciple was Gahaninath, whose disciple was Nivrittinath, who was the Guru of Gyannath. Therefore his teachings are very much of the *Nath* lineage, even to contemporary Yoga practitioners. He authored *Amrita Anubhava* (Experience of Immortality), which shows his spiritual roots lie in the teachings of Gorakshanath, a living embodiment of immortality and an incarnation of Shi*va* himself. His philosophical stance was *Sphurti Vada*, understood as the doctrine of spontaneous manifestation. He believed deeply in the excellence of the *Nath Yoga* doctrine which added *bhakti* or devotion instilled with wisdom—it was to him a composite whole.

The Lord Jnaneswar has extolled Yoga as the supreme path to Self-Realization. At the same time he understood that the most excellent of these Yoga practices were not possible for the simple and common masses to perform. So, out of his compassion, he encouraged and showed the people the path of devotion (*bhakti*). This later took the form of the *bhakti* movement in Maharashtra state. The masses who embraced this movement were called the "*Varkaris*". The path of devotion, although slower than the classic yogic path, is nonetheless easier, and more people tend to be attracted to devotional chanting.

Of course, it is best to combine both Yoga and devotion for the optimum spiritual progress.

When Jnaneswar was a child of twelve years, he was being ridiculed and doubted by society and the people of his village concerning his spiritual yogic practices and powers. Now during those times, there lived a great Nath Yogi called Chandeva, and he, having heard of the harassment to little Jnannath, went to bless and to certify the boy saint's spiritual status. The Nath Chandeva, is said to have then been over fourteen hundred years old and since he had no enemies in the world, the wild beasts of the jungles served him. He rode on a tiger to meet Jnannath and his family. Upon seeing him, the villagers were terrified but he told them to be calm. The great Chandeva told the people that Jnannath was a true son of God and a Nath Yogi and then blessed the whole village. The Nath Chandeva raised the kundalini power latent in Jnannath, which made the wall on which Jnannath and his brothers and sister were sitting move. This convinced the doubting villagers of Alandi as to the spiritual prowess of Jnannath. Then Chandeva, having blessed the village, left for his jungle abode near the town which is today called Saswad.

It is ironic that in medieval times, due to the ignorance of the Nath Yogic tradition among the masses, some fanatic cults of the bhakti movement tried to belittle and falsify the spiritual stature of the lofty Nath Chandeva. This was irresponsible jargon by partisan cultists. The yogi must be seen in his proper perspective. Jnaneswar never ceased to extol the excellence of Yoga and gave *bhakti* to the masses out of compassion.

I belong to the same yogic family lineage of Babaji-Gorakshanath and therefore to Jnannath. My family members were the traditional governors of Pune district even at that time, and the responsibility of good governance fell upon us. As time went by, well after the *mahasamadhi* of Jnannath, his annual celebratory procession was taken out into the streets. As the governors and chiefs of the land (*Deshmukhs*), my family was bound to provide protection to the *palkhi* (palanquin) in which Jnannath's silver sandals were installed. So even today, one of our junior family's horses heads the sacred procession of Jnaneswar's palanquin. Then, the senior family to which I belong, ties the ceremonial gold brocade turban on the image of Jnannath. Then only, when we raise the saffron flag on top of the temple, does the sacred procession begin.

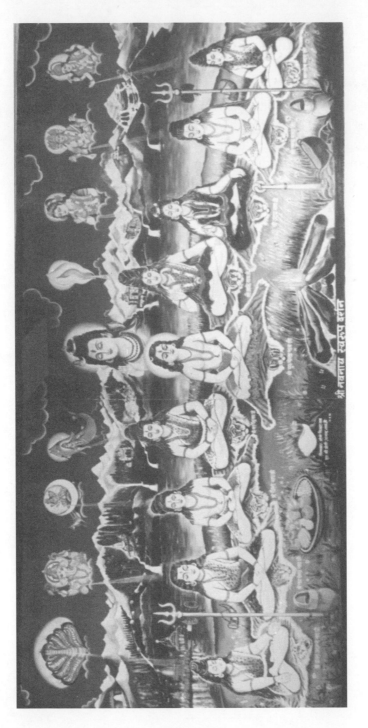

The Celestial Hierarchy of the Nine Naths

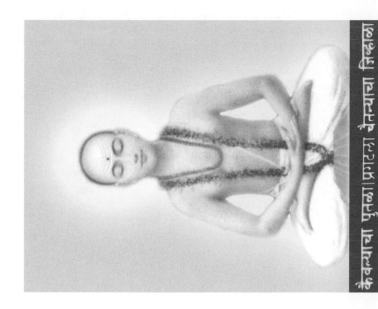

केवल्याचा पूर्तल (प्रतल्ल) चेतन्याचा सिद्धळ

Babaji Gorakshanath's disciple Gyanath
St. Gyaneshwar (Lord of Wisdom) of the yogic
family lineage of Yogiraj Gurunath

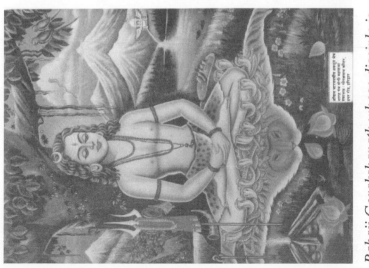

Babaji Gorakshanath whose disciple is
Gahaninath whose disciple Nivruttinath
whose disciple is Gyannath

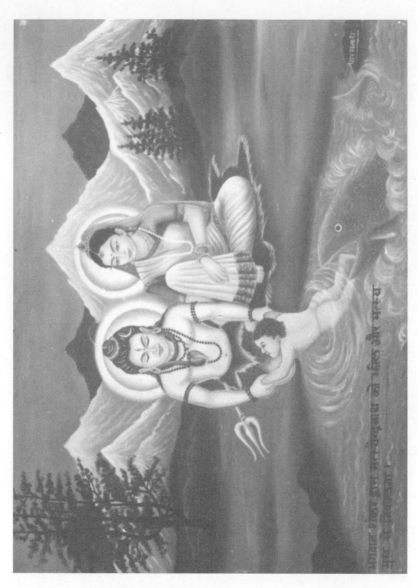

Lord Shiva teaches Yoga to Matsyendranath

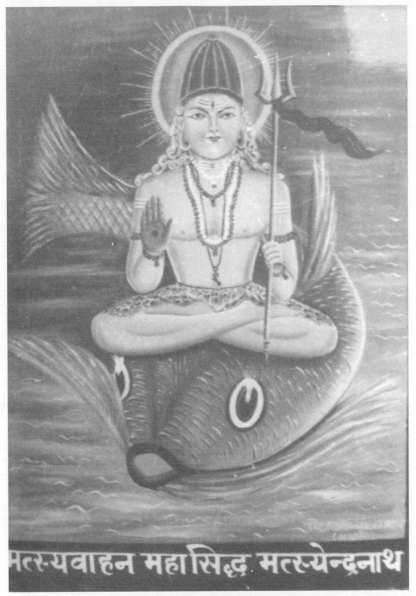

मत्स्यवाहन महासिद्ध मत्स्येन्द्रनाथ

Yogeshwar Matsyendranath
The founder of Kaula Tradition, Shabari Vidya and Tantra Yoga.
Known as Avalokiteshwara in Buddhist Tradition
The disciple of Shiva-Goraksha-Babaji on the divine plane and
His Guru on the earthly plane. This is the Leela (Divine Play).

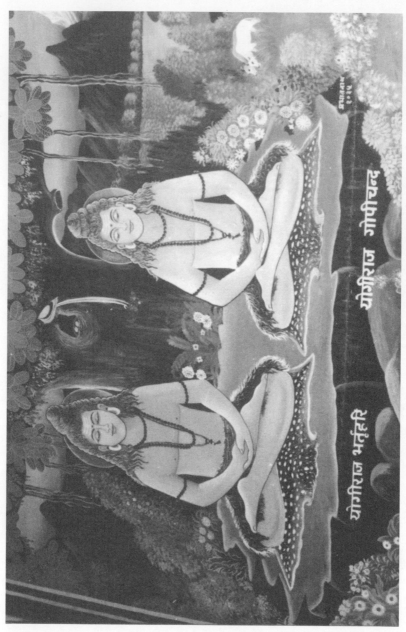

योगिराज भर्तृहरि   योगिराज गोपीचन्द्

Yogiraj Bhartrinath and Yogiraj Gopichand

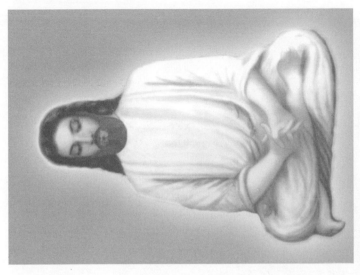

Jesus (Isha Nath) learned the science of yoga and immortality from Chetan Nath of the mystical order of Goraknathis

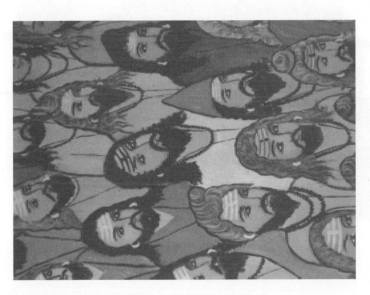

Jesus (Isha Nath) with the Nath Yogis
Photo: Gorakshanath Ashram, Haradwar

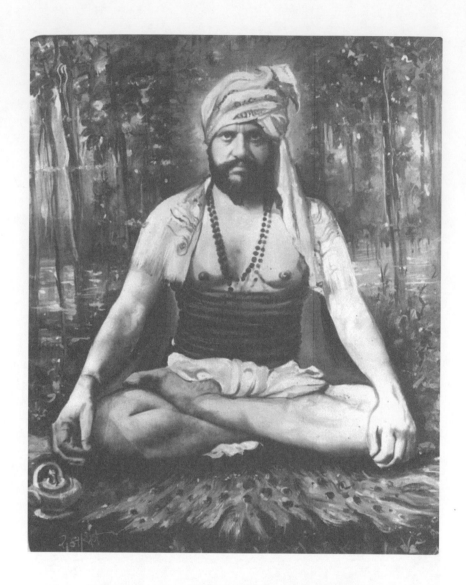

Yogiraj Gurunath Siddhanath in Nath Regalia

CHAPTER 10

THE NATH SIDDHA TRADITION

During my travels to *ashrams*, through jungles, and to the Himalayas, I interacted with the whole cross-section of saints, yogis and spiritual masters of India. Amongst them I found the contribution of the *Nath Yogis* to the spiritual legacy of India to be the most remarkable, particularly concerning *Raja* and *Hatha Yoga*. The *Nath Yogis* are the greatest *Hatha* and *Raja* yogis that ever walked the earth and are no doubt the authorities on the subject of rejuvenation and *Kaya Kalpa*. It was to these forms of *yogic* practice and philosophy that I was most drawn.

Traditionally there are eighty-four *Siddhas*, and over and above them, nine *Mahasiddhas* called the *Nava-Naths*. The term *Siddha* means a perfected being who is totally liberated from *samsara* (the world wheel which turns by the power of ignorance). They are adepts who, having transcended the fifth degree of initiation, have moved up the evolutionary ladder and expanded to serve humanity as their larger Self. The nine *Mahasiddhas* are those adepts who have achieved the seventh degree of initiation and beyond to the eighth and ninth degree of divine Is-ness. More will be revealed about them in the next chapter.

The *Siddhas* and their *sangh* are the core foundation of the systems of Yoga and *yogachara* (yoga teaching). Their ways of yoga are pre-*vedic*, antedating Buddhism, Jainism and even Hinduism. Gautama, who later became the enlightened Buddha, not only learned from them but he was also one of them. He later went on to found his own school and philosophy, born of the ancient *Siddha* and *Nath* tradition. Such also was the case of the great Mahavira (a

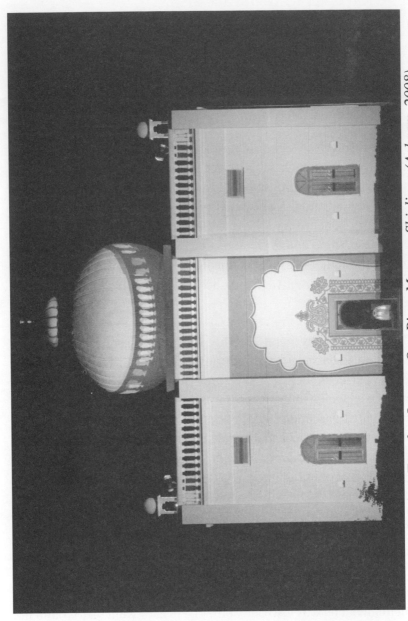

Earth Peace Temple - Largest One Piece Mercury Shivlinga (Ashram, 2008)

contemporary of Buddha, who expounded the Jain philosophy). His followers then had two subsects called the Shvetambars and the Digambars

The *Siddhas* may choose their dwellings at will, roaming the cities like the Siddha Trilanga Swami who resided at Manikarnika Ghat in Varanasi. However, they are mostly found in the Himalayan ranges, silent and away from public gaze, as in the case of *Siddha-Avadhoot* Raja Sundernath who chooses the snowy abode of Alkapuri beyond Badrinath. They are the guardians of the Himalayan peaks, established in *sanjeevani samadhi* for thousands of years in undecayable bodies of light for the salvation of the world.

In their selfless service, the *Siddhas* and *Mahasiddhas* (the nine *Naths*), form what is known as The Guardian Wall of Humanity. They have denied themselves the highest state of salvation, remaining incarnate until the time their lesser brothers come to Self-realization. Their Great Spirit permeates the evolutionary impulse of humanity and their force drives our infant race along its evolutionary journey towards divinity.

The Scope and Sweep of Yoga

There never has been, nor will there ever be a time when man's own nature shall cease to demand its best and foremost attention to unraveling the Truth. Yoga is the most excellent way of doing so, commending itself to the foremost minds of the east and the west. Men of marvelous mental power and intense heroism of ancient India were the outcome of the teachings of Yoga.

It is true that Yoga is the science of all sciences because it deals with the very essence of the evolution and well being of humanity. It is the one and only science offering the knowledge and practice of total transformation. This is the transformation from man the brute, to man the man, to man the God. It is for this reason that the supreme love, the love for the divine and love for humanity, may be experienced through yoga.

Yoga Philosophy in Nath Parampara (tradition)

The basic Indian philosophy of *samsara* is that this world is a wheel of time (*kala chakra*) that rotates due to spiritual ignorance (*avidya*). Its six spokes are virtue (*dharma*), vice (*adharma*), pleasure (*sukha*), pain (*dukha*), attachment (*raga*), and aversion (*dvesha*). These qualities are the cause of *karma* (cause and effect) and subsequently *punarjanma* (cycle of birth and death). The objective of yoga in the *Nath* tradition is to become a *jivan mukta* (liberated soul), completely free from *samsara*, the cycle of birth and death (*punarjanma*), while living.

In nature, the yogi perceives a single force working in two directions. From the outer objective it struggles to separate, but from the inner it struggles to unite. The inner force is called life while the outer force is called death. The purpose of Yoga is to unite life with death.

The yogis are aware that all in the manifest (*vyakta*) and unmanifest (*avyakta*) universe comes from the same primordial source of divine intelligence. And more than this, the yogis are aware that individual consciousness is part and parcel of the Universal Consciousness. Man is a mere spark of this unfathomable Truth.

But so involved is one in matter, time, and space that the individual loses all recognition of his or her true identity. The soul becomes so involved in the enjoyment of sensory pleasures and lust for life in matter that it mistakes itself for the ego covering and its sensual mind. We say that one's true identity is covered by the veil of *maya*, matter swayed by attraction (*raga*) and repulsion (*dvesha*).

The school of the *Nath* tradition sets forth a means and a way of life for bringing the individual soul back to its true and original position, absolving it from every aspect of causation, space and time. Through the process of Yoga the individual consciousness gains control and ultimately becomes one with the universal spirit, the source of its true Being. The yogi becomes a *jivan mukta*, free from all *karma*, and enters *Brahma nirvana*, the God-essence. He reclaims his lost birthright as the son of Divine Truth by losing his false ego identity and merging into the divine, whereby he may partake of this unlimited consciousness of Truth, which is all love, all wisdom, and all power.

Nath Parampara and Samkhya

The *Nath* philosophy of yoga sets forth the same cosmological doctrine that is set forth in the *Samkhya* tradition. *Samkhya* is primarily concerned with the universal condition of nature and Yoga pertains to the individual condition of consciousness. Both are based on the fundamental logical premise that something cannot come out of nothing. Every shadow must have its substance. Life proceeds from life just as light proceeds from light and not darkness. Likewise, the yogic system says that the gross individual must have a divine consciousness from which he manifests himself and to which he will return.

The force called life unites spirit and matter to bring all things into being. Man is the offspring of the whole invisible form of nature appearing when his *karma* is ripe through the phenomenon of birth, the physical manifestation of an individual aspect of the universal consciousness. Therefore the soul (*Jiva*) co-operates in both the subjective and objective worlds. Mortal man, being a compound entity, has the inherent quality of dissolution. However, he is made up of both the mortal and the immortal. The former is known by the senses, but the subtle soul is known only by spiritual perception and realized by the practice of Yoga.

The Sum and Substance of Man

Man is a combination of consciousness and five elements of matter (*bhutas*). His soul is ever evolving into a body of matter through the dynamics of the combined sperm and ovum. The soul is potentially present as the essence of knowingness. Only when by yogic meditation one realizes himself is he expressed as the "Lightless Light of Knowingness".

The Soul or individual spirit is called Jiva. This term is derived from the Sanskrit root *jiv* "to live". It is the individual soul, the spark of life within each of us, the animating principle of one's true being, the feeling of a constant witness in a fleeting world. It cannot be seen but only experienced. The *Jiva* is a spark of the universal soul known as *Purusha* in *Samkhya*. So we have the universal spirit (*Purusha*) as the core subjective aspect of nature (*Prakriti*) and the soul (*Jiva*) as the subjective aspect of the individual in this phenomenal world.

In the universal condition of nature, the cosmic substance (*Prakriti*), consists of three sub automic qualities or constituents called *gunas*. They are: *sattva* (luminosity), *rajas* (activity), and *tamas* (inertia). Their function in the universal condition of nature is to reveal, to activate/to move, and to restrain, respectively. In the phenomenal world, due to their intricate intercourse, they signify adhesion, cohesion, and disintegration. An individual who is born of nature possesses the three *gunas* in varying degrees. *Sattva guna* gives happiness, *rajas* moves to action, and *tamas* breeds indolence and heedlessness.

The subtle body or *linga sharir*, also called the *linga deha*, is that which serves the soul (*Jiva*) as its vehicle and survives the destruction of the physical body. It is constant and does not change through the cycles of life and death. However, it is not eternal and is reabsorbed into the elements of which it is composed when the soul is liberated from body and mind.

The Gross Body is the material perishable body called the *sthula sharir*, which is destroyed at death while the soul (*jiva*) reincarnates into another form at birth. The gross body is composed of five *bhutas* or elements known as the *pancha mahabhuti sharir*.

The *linga sharir* is composed of eighteen elements. They are: intelligence (*buddhi*), ego (*ahamkara*), mind (*manas*), the five knowing senses (*jnanendriyas*), the five working senses (*karmendriyas*) and the five subtle elements (*tanmatras*). All this is the sum and substance of man.

In order to understand the eighteen elements we must also understand the indivisual collective mind or *chitta*. When the word *chitta* is used for the mind, it refers to the entire knowing faculty, "mind" in a collective sense. Another term used for mind is *antakarna* meaning "the inner doing" or "doer". It is the internal faculty or organ, the seat of thought and feeling. Patanjali speaks of the necessity for the total restrain of this function in his treatise *The Yoga Sutras*.

The mind-*chitta* is the first manifestation in the world of name and form. It is the first birth of consciousness manifesting itself with one's first breath of life. Its distinguishing feature is awareness and it has the capacity to know and influence its environment. The mind-*chitta's* processes are divided into two general subsections: conscious behavior and unconscious behavior.

Consciousness is a characteristic of any organic creature that is receiving impressions or having experience. Conscious behavior consists of all processes of sensation and feeling of which an individual is aware. Unconscious behavior consists of the subconscious experiences and impressions of the individual that are neither felt nor experienced by the conscious mind, unaware of what is happening around it.

Mind-*chitta* is further divided into three categories in accordance with the three functions of the conscious and unconscious mental processes. They are: intelligence (*buddhi*), ego (*ahamkara*), and mind (*manas*). Each has its distinguishing characteristics and individual functions but are the same unit and form one working whole.

The first stage of the synthetic unit called *chitta*-mind is the intellect or *buddhi* derived from *Budh* - "to wake up, recover consciousness, observe". Here it is used to mean the seat of intelligence, non-attachment, wisdom and virtue. It is the intuitive capacity of the individual for direct perception. *Buddhi* manifests through determination, resolution in thought and action, and retention of concepts and values. It is the last action in the mental process. It is the mere awareness without thought of "I". *Manasi* raises the objects of thoughts and *buddhi* dwells upon them (*sadsatvivek buddhi*).

The ego or "I maker" is called *Ahamkara*. It is the second stage of the *chitta*-mind. It is the vast reservoir of instinctive impulses dominated by pleasure, pain, and blind impulsive wishing. It is the arrogating principle of "I know", "I exist", and "I have", the basis of ideation and self-identity however much subdued and indistinct. It arrogates to itself the experiences of the mind (*manas*) and passes it on to the intelligence (*buddhi*) to be dwelled upon and determined. This aspect of mind causes oneself to identify as a body, the heresy of mistaken identity. This is the individualized self.

The little Mind or *manas* is the third stage of the synthetic unit called *chitta*-mind. It constitutes the group of cognitive processes responsible for rationalization. It is the material force that obscures Consciousness. *Manas* is the seat of all desire, of thought, rationalization, idealism, affection, mood swings and temper. The capacity for thinking is an internal quality of its nature that never ceases. It is the power behind all action functioning in association with the knowing senses (*jnanendriyas*) and the working senses (*karmendriyas*). It has the capacity of selection, rejection and attention yet it is unable to reveal itself to the one who is experiencing. It can perceive but can not conceive like *buddhi*. It is merely the instrument through which thoughts enter, the collective organ of sensation, the sensorium.

In relation to the external world,
the mind – manasi perceives and presents,
the Ego – ahamkara arrogates,
the intelligence – buddhi discriminates, decides and acts.

The subtle elements or *tanmatras* are formed in the next stage in the integration of a being. It is the manifestation of the five rudiments of matter, the subtle elements (*tanmatras*). They are the ethereal essence of sound (*sabda*), touch (*sparsa*), form (*rupa*), flavor (*rasa*), and odor (*gandha*). These elements can not be apprehended by the gross senses but by intuition only. The subtle forms of matter (*tanmatra*) are referred to as mere dream stuff. They manifest themselves to the mind as lights during *yoni mudra* (an advanced yogic process.) This is the mind-stuff of the subtle body not yet materialized.

The group of subtle Senses or *indriyas* is the next stage in the making of man which consists of the knowing senses (*jnanendriyas*) and working senses (*karmendriyas*). The *indriyas* (sense powers) comprise the sense consciousness through which the mind receives all its impressions from the objective world. The knowing senses are the powers to hear, feel, see, taste and smell. They function through their respective organs, the ears, skin, eyes, tongue and nose.

The working senses are the powers to express (*vak*), grasp (*pani*), move (*pada*), procreate (*upashta*), and excrete (*payu*). All sense *indriyas* constitute the awareness of the response which the lower mind (*manasi*) makes to the objects presented by those senses. The *indriyas* are the means whereby enjoyment is had which is the will to live.

The elements of Nature or *bhutas* form the last stage in the manifestation of a being. It is the appearance of the five gross elements (*bhutas*) as perceived by the senses. They are: ether (*akasha*), air (*vayu*), fire (*agni*), water (*apas*), and earth (*prithivi*). The five gross elements are the result of the aggregation of the subtle elements (*tanmatras*). This is what we may call mind-stuff materialized. The gross *bhutas* come into being as a result of the slowing down of the more subtle aspects of nature.

Each of the grosser elements (*bhutas*) evolves out of its subtler element (*tanmatras*). Sound creates for its vehicle the homogenous unit of ether. Touch creates the vehicle of air next and then form (*rupa*) creates fire (*agni*). The next evolution is water, the vehicle of flavor (*rasa*) and the last evolution to manifest itself in nature is earth (*prithivi*), vehicle of odor (*gandha*), the lowest vibration of nature.

The five forms of gross matter are transformed states of original nature characterized by their qualities (*gunas*) of *satva*, *rajas*, and *tamas* as are all material things animate and inanimate. The physical body of man is formed by the union of man's sperm and woman's ova to become the body formed of food, the *sthula sharir* or *annamayee kosha*.

A Synopsis of Yoga

Yoga is the practice of absorption of Soul into Spirit
whereby
Sorrow and Desire creating Karma dissolve
consequently,
Freeing one's soul bound to the Cycle of Birth and Death
giving it
The Final Liberation – Niranjana – Nirvana

Path of Achievement

Hatha Yoga

1. *Asana*: Bodily postures for strength and health (*maha-mudra, khechari mudra, yoni mudra*).

2. *Pranayama*: Cleansing of *nadis* (the 72,000 psychic nerves) and the raising of the *pranic Kundalini* in the *sushumna nadi*.

3. *Pratyahara*: Withdrawal of *prana* from the five senses (*indriyas*) and the withdrawal of the electric flow of *prana, ojas*, and *tejas* from the 72,000 psychic nerves (*nadis*) to the navel (*kanda*) (by the processes of *vajroli, sahajoli*, and *amaroli*).

Raja Yoga

4. *Dharana* (*manas*): Concentration of the *pranic kundalini* in the spine (*sushumna nadi*) causing it to pierce the six lotuses (*chakras*) and three *granthis* or psychic locks.

5. *Dhyana* (*buddhi*): *Dhyana* occurs when the *kundalini* enters the third ventricle of the brain known as The Cave of Brahma. Here

Kundalini (Shakti) resides with Shiva in *sabikalpa samadhi* as The *Hamsa* Soul.

6. *Samadhi* (*Atman*): As The *Hamsa* Soul, the *kundalini* energy ascends to the lateral ventricles of the brain to win her wings to freedom. Here she resides as the *Paramhansa* in *nirvikalpa samadhi*, at one with her Lord *Shiva*.

7. *Divya deha*: An immaculate body of rainbow colored light free from the ravages of time, for uninterrupted communion with God. The divine radiant body is created by *Sanjeevani Yoga* involving yogic ingestion of mercury, *pranayama*, proper diet and God's grace.

Hatha-Raja Yoga

There can be no Raja Yoga without Hatha Yoga
Just as there can be no butter without milk.

The *Hatha-Raja* yogi, with his body of radiant light in his divine realization, meets the *Raja* yogi at the same level of consciousness. The apparent detour of the *Hatha* yogi's *kundalini* practice is not futile for he acquires a total transformation of his body-mind-soul. He does not view Self-realization as an event separate from life in the physical realm. Hence the realization of the *Hatha* yogi is in fact more complete than that of the *Raja* yogi for the simple reason that it includes the radiant body of immortality.

I would strongly advocate the practice of Yoga along the course of *Hatha-Raja-Yoga* rather than *Raja Yoga* alone. The latter would be like setting out for the Ph.D. degree without comprehending the preliminary levels of study. The yogi must practice *Hatha Yoga* to the extent he can and get as much body fitness and health as possible. I know it's not possible for all aspirants to acquire the radiant body, but we can get a partial radiant body and mind. To neglect the needs of bodily health is to falsify the eternal doctrine of the unity of all and the divinity of all. Governed by the philosophy of "*All is Brahman*," even the simplest of needs and actions take on a divine significance. It is Shakti who sees and hears and enjoys through our body temple, which is Her manifestation, housing Him, the Divine Indweller.

The *Hatha-Raja Yoga* system of Gorakshanath holds, within its power, humanity's hope for physical immortality combined with divine liberation. The tradition of *Hatha Yoga* has an immense wealth of hard won gold, information about the potentials of body and mind. Modern medicine, psychology, and advanced scientific methods are rediscovering some amazing facts that the *Nath* yogis have taught and demonstrated in their lives for thousands of years.

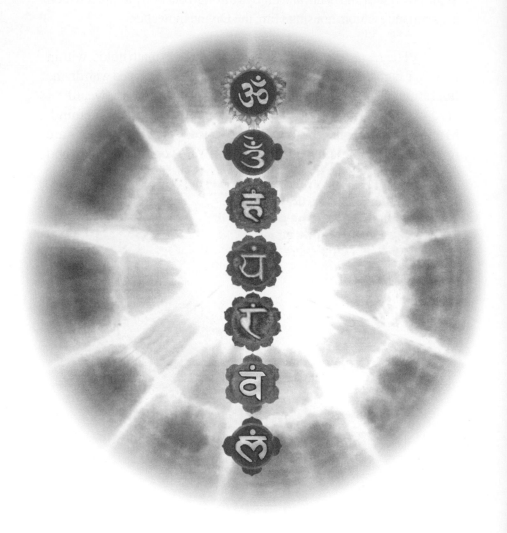

Individual and Cosmic Chakras

CHAPTER 11

INDIVIDUAL & COSMIC CHAKRAS

Karma is Samsara, Yoga is Moksha

Soul is bound to Samsara by
Karmic cycle of birth and death
Yoga transforms Karma
Liberates you to Moksha.

From the ancient of days the yogis discovered in their bodies the seven basic *chakras*. They are the vital shrines that are spiritually awakened by the Divine *Kundalini*. Upon awakening them, the negative blocks that impede one's evolutionary path to enlightenment are removed. The *chakras* were known to the great *Nath Yogis* of the Himalayas who used this knowledge for purely spiritual purposes and only rarely to strike at the vital centers in self-defense.

The sacred art of *marmasthan chakra* (vital center) was later taught to the Tibetan Buddhist monks who also made use of these vital strike centers for spiritual and psychic purposes. *Padmasambhava* took this science from India to Tibet. The Tibetan Buddhists then brought this knowledge to the Chinese who used this science for psychic and therapeutic purposes.

There is evidence to show that the martial arts originated in India and were later given to Tibetan monks who took and taught it to the Chinese. The great Bodhidharma from South India was the supreme teacher at the temple of Shaolin in China where he taught them the martial arts known in *Sanskrit* as *Kara Hati* (to do with hands) and *Varmannie*.

From China, the cultural migration of the knowledge of *chakras* went to Japan where the Japanese used these vital *Marma* points as martial arts striking points in Indo and Karate. Their *Atemiwaza* striking points are the locations taken from the *chakras* in the Indian Yoga system.

Destiny in Your Chakras

The *chakras* are vortices of *pranic* energy vibrations and are the storehouses of our past, present, and future *karma*. By the science of *Kundalini Kriya Yoga*, *Mantra Yoga*, and *pranayama*, the yogi may transform his *karmic* limitations and speed up his evolution to merge with the Divine, *Brahma Nirvana*. As I focused on my *chakras* during my meditation practice, their energy patterns flowed more smoothly. I experienced great ease and order in my meditative lifestyle. As I progressed in my *sadhana*, I realized that my destiny was determined by the vibration energy patterns of my *chakras*.

Not only do *pranic* vibrations form the petals of the *chakras*, but each *chakra* also emits a resonance frequency, a seed sound vibration called *beej mantra*. These sounds are given in the classic Yoga texts. I applied them to each *chakra* during my meditation, and there were wonderful effects in relation to my health and tranquility of mind. This practice is called "Internal *Chakra Dharana*," also known as "*Kundalini* Awakening" and involves advanced yogic methods.

I must caution against the untutored chanting of *mantras* by my western brothers and sisters. A slight error in the speech vibration of the *mantra* could change the meaning, the texture, and the ultimate result of the *mantra*. This would then not resolve the problem or achieve the goal for which the practice is performed. It would be wise for new-age students and western teachers to learn the Sanskrit phonetics from an Indian Master or Sanskrit scholar and not a Buddhist or Japanese teacher.*

Karma Deposited in Your Chakras

My fascination with the *Kundalini* energy rising up the spine to penetrate the *chakras* was a profound experience for me. This led me into a meditative exploration in the laboratory of my subtle bodies. Persevering in practice, I began to realize that both positive and negative *karmas* were lodged as vibrations in my *astral chakras*. From there they were transferred to the *pranic chakras* and then to the nitrogen nubs of the genes to be worked out through my mind, my physical body, and my circumstances.

The nitrogen nubs of all human genes are composed of magnetic vibrations that synchronize with the vibrations of *pranic chakras* and subsequently record our past *karma* that is to be played out in this life-drama. As the body inhabited by our soul grows, vibrations of resonant thought (*nama*) recorded in the tape of our genetic nubs begin to take form (*rupa*) and materialize as good or bad attitudes and circumstantial *karma*. This process of expansion of the *karmic* web influences our lifestyle, our behavioral attitudes, as well as our whole personality. The circumstances we are governed by are *karmicly* influenced by what we have brought upon ourselves due to past deeds.

---

*A special caution must be maintained while chanting *mantras*. Learning from a book could be quite misleading as far as pronunciations are concerned. In a market inundated with New Age Yoga books written by people not trained in India and having no knowledge of Sanskrit, pronunciation errors can occur in intonation of *mantras* like the *Gayatri, the Mrytunjaya, beej* and *mula mantras,* which could have *karmic* consequences.

I therefore combined my meditations with outer investigations by meeting with other *yogis* and reading the relevant books on the subject. I knew then that I had done the exercises before.

Our *Karma* is Encoded in Our DNA

Karmas are a carry over of our past deeds of right and wrong. They lie latent in our personal *akashic* records of radiant light. When the soul incarnates into the womb of its mother, its past, as radiant tape recordings, enters the etheric mold of the embryo to be later impressed and decoded as thought vibrations on the nitrogen nubs of its DNA. Our good and bad deeds encoded in the DNA of our *pranic chakras* mark their time until the opportune moments and circumstances offer themselves and allow the ripened *karma* to fructify. They are, we could say, like timed release photons. Only then do our DNA *karmas* express themselves to actualize into action, emotion, or meditative practices.

Nullifying Karma by Kundalini and Mantra Yoga

Karmas, both good and bad, are latent in our *chakras* as resonant thoughts. The *Kundalini* is light, sound, and vibration. The *mantras* are also sound vibrations. By synchronizing the appropriate *mantra* sound with the resonant thoughts of *karma* in a *chakra*, one's accumulated *karma* can be resolved, transformed, or nullified by playing the *mantric* vibration against the *karmic* vibration. Instead of waiting for negative *karma* to manifest, an individual may resolve *karma* by working directly to release, nullify, or transform the *karmic* energy patterns latent in his or her *chakras*.

We are using these *chakras* for the ultimate healing, called enlightenment, which is originally what the *Nath Yogis* intended them to be used for. As the *Kundalini* rises up the spine, She is associated with the sounds of *Lam, Vung, Ram, Yum, Ha*, and *Aum* at the six stations of *pranic* vibration. At each center, she dissolves and transforms our *karma* to give us enlightenment. This is known to be the Supreme Healing, to be one with God - what more could one desire?

Cosmic Man: Unfolding of the Septenary Man

There are seven cosmic beings known as the *Sapta Rishis*, the seven primeval sages of our galaxy. They are our *Ishvars* and informing spirits. *Ishvars* are secondary gods below Parameshwar, the Lord God. Their biographies are not only written in the *akashic* records, but they are also written in the ancient archives of India, the great libraries of the Himalayas.

The *Rishis* are those great cosmic beings like Vashishta and Vishwamitra who came during the Lemurian times, the Atlantean times, and the early Aryan times, where Lord Rama prevailed as the *avatara* of Vishnu. There were two *gurus* teaching him. One was the *Rishi* Vashishta, his family guru, who wrote the treatise called the Yoga Vashishta. Then we have the other guru, Vishwamitra, who taught Rama the life supporting and liberating *Gayatri Mantra*. He also taught him the art of self-defense and noble warfare.

The Seven Great Sages are the informing spirits of the seven stars of the *Sapta Rishi* Constellation (the Great Bear constellation).* Have you ever seen, on a clear night, the stars of the Great Bear?

---

*Mysteriously, the *Rishis* of the Great Bear are connected with a form of *Shiva Vastuspati*, the hunter *Vyad*, which the Egyptians later called the Dog Star. The "*Mrug Nakshatra*", the deer - later called Orion in the west - is hunted by the Great Hunter—*Vastuspati Shiva*. From Him sprang all the *Vastushastra*, the essence of geomancy, later influencing heavily the Chinese science *Feng Shui*.

They're now known as Cannis Major. But this is recent information that the west has brought. From ancient days the Seven Primeval Sages were known as the *Sapta Rishi*. The first is Marichi, then Atri and Pulastya, then Pulaha, Angiras, Vashishta and Vishwamitra.

Now every human being is astrologically connected to one of these Seven Primeval Sages who are our living Gods. My *gotra*, for instance, is the last but one called Vashishta. We call it a *gotra*, that is, your spiritual ancestry, source and origin. It traces up to one of these seven stars.

If you look very carefully in the night sky near the last but one star of the Great Bear called sage Vashishta you will see another little star by its side. She is Arundhati, his faithful wife. She stayed by the side of the great Master Vashishta, always and eternally a symbol of loyalty to her husband. The other wives left their sages in order to nurture and bring up the great child of Shiva called Kartikeya. A cluster of stars is also seen in the night and they are called the *Krittika*, the six wives of the *Rishis* of the Great Bear.

Whenever in India a marriage ceremony takes place, the husband will take the wife out under the evening sky and he points to Arundhati. He points to the faithful wife and she points also. They are supposed to point hand in hand. This shows the eternal faithfulness with which the marriage is solemnized. That's why in India you see that very rarely do marriages break. They continue how many years? For thirty years, forty years, fifty years, they are married. It all goes on, smiles and quarrels and laughter and crying but they still stay together because it's a solemn oath.

So they say, be faithful like Arundhati. Be faithful. So she is ever shining by her Lord Vashishta, the primeval Sage. I've gone a bit off track here because I thought this may be of interest to you. It's a part of Indian culture you see. Besides, when the husband is there with his newly wed beautiful wife, he likes to get close to her. So he stands and then puts his hand on top of her hand and he points to

Arundhati. That's part of the romance, but the spirit behind this ritual is faithfulness.

Now our seven chakra centers are connected to the seven major planets of our solar system, which are guiding principles. Those seven planets of the solar system are the seven *chakras* of the Solar Man with the sun as its main spiritual center. Those *chakras* in the planetary network are further connected to a larger cosmic man whose *chakras* are the stars of the Great Bear constellation. Each of these stars is hundreds of thousands of time bigger than our sun, almost as big as our whole solar system. So if one of the stars of the Great Bear had to replace the sun, its belly would graze the Earth and our Earth would evaporate.

The star sages of the Great Bear, called the *Sapta Rishi*, connect themselves to the seven galaxies of our cluster. Each of the seven galaxies is a *chakra* in the body of the God called *Swayambhu Manu*. Each galaxy is a hundred thousand light years across. So, if you were to measure it at the speed of light, it would take a hundred thousand years for the light to travel from one tip of the galaxy to the other tip of the galaxy.

Now there are millions of galaxies in a cluster. But these seven galaxies are the ancient ones and directly connect to the seven clusters. Each of these clusters is six trillion light years across, and forms one *chakra* in the body of Brahma. These seven clusters connect to the seven super-clusters, each of which forms a lotus of the Preserver called Lord Vishnu (God, the Christos). Then these seven super-clusters connect to the seven universes. These primeval universes are the *chakra* lotuses of the body of Lord Shiva, "He About Whom Naught May Be Said". And then the seven complete universes connect to the seven infinities. Those seven infinities connect to infinite infinities of "Him About Whom We Know Nothing".

Who knows and who doesn't know—who knows? Therefore it is best to fall into silence and humble ourselves at the feet of man and God because humility is the best way. That's right, and this is the reason I deliberately took you on this beautiful spiritual surfing on the high seas of the cosmos to show you how lost we would be and how little we are and what a good reason we have to be humble. Where is our knowledge and where is what we learn? Where are we? Nowhere. Nothing. Only the Absolute is!

The Healing Process

As far as the healing process goes, Masters are working in a particular way. When they do healing or when they do work for humanity what is happening spiritually is that they are working through certain light connections, like optic fibers, filaments. These tubes, which are like photonic tunnels of light, connect the seven *chakras* of the disciple to the seven *chakras* of the *Satguru*. From the physical, the light connections go to the astral, then to the causal and the spiritual. The Master works through these light tubes in the astral and the mental and then on to the causal where all our *karma* is lodged.

The planets are connected to the seven centers of the *Satguru* by similar astral and spiritual tubes of light. They are photons of light, which lengthen like optic fibers, only these spiritual optic fibers are made of the ruby flash or emerald flash, or the blue sapphire flash. These are healing and evolving energies connected with the seven planets.

Each planet is in itself a *chakra* of the solar system man, with the seven planetary *chakras* connecting with the seven *chakras* of the Great Bear, the *Sapta Rishi*. From there the energies or the "informing spirits" of those centers enter through the vortices of the planetary *chakras* until they come to the *chakras* of the *Satguru*. The *Satguru* pulls out through the negative tubes all of the disciple's negativity, all his

206

evil *karma*. The Guru withdraws the disciple's *karma* through his *chakras* and passes it on into the whirlpool of planets in the healing process.

All this healing operates like the circulatory system with the heart as its pump. The Guru pumps his life's fresh blood, his fresh *prana*, fresh oxygen into the disciple from *chakra* to *chakra*, into whichever center the disciple needs. He withdraws the disciple's negativity into himself, into his own body, from the physical, mental, and emotional bodies. He withdraws the negativities from the disciple's body and suffers them or transforms them into nectar in his own body, if he can. Otherwise he passes them on to the seven planets and then to the Seven Rishis, the *Gotrabhus* (the seven stars of the Great Bear).

Who is healing? And who is making the sacrifices? It is the Guardian Spirits of Humanity, the great *Maha Siddhas*, but they choose to heal not the physical body, which is the apparent self. They emphasize the healing of one's true Self, the Soul, and that barrier that blocks the expression of the Self, that is, the barrier of negative mind. That is what is diseased and is caught like a lichen under your consciousness. Therefore, what we yogis heal is not the physical body, but we heal any disease which is obstructing one's spiritual expression, and that is the negative mind.

In the Declaration of Human Rights for Earth Peace, I have said, "Allow yourself to heal and to be healed." But from what? From the negativity of the mind! How? By letting go of the negative mind. Very simple! My healing as the *Satguru*, or the Master, or the Rabbi, has to do with the negative mind. If the negative mind is healed and dissolved, then all physical disease will automatically go. This is my experience. Now, contemporary medicine agrees with ancient Yoga that practically all diseases are psychosomatic. The negative mind is their source of origin.

You can't give the physical body more importance than the Self Soul. The apparent self is not more important than the real Self.

Give the physical body secondary importance. Spiritual Knowledge or *Atma Vidya* and healing of the negativity of the mind have more importance than the healing of the body! And how may we heal the negativity of the mind? By certain yogic techniques and *pranayama* methods. The direct method is the stilling of the mind of the student by the Master.

When the Master gives the "Here Now" experience there is no thought and there is no negativity. When there is no negativity, there is no filter of venous blood in the system. The Master works the spiritual heart of the disciples. He pumps the fresh *prana* into the seven *chakras* of the disciples and takes their venous *prana* into his own Being. He is therefore giving his life's blood to cure the disciple of the negativity of his mind. Physical problems also get cured as a secondary effect. If I say, "*Alakh Niranjan*" and one person's headaches goes and another's ulcers are also cured, then what can I do? It's just overflow of the Master's spiritual healing energy.

Healers are very much into the intellectual splitting of hairs. What is the use of the splitting of hair if you can't control the hare of your own mind? The hare is darting hither and thither like a wild rabbit and you are going on a wild goose chase trying to control your own thoughts. The relationship between the healer and the to-be healed requires the healer to control his own thoughts. This is something the majority of healers cannot do.

So, with an untrained mind and only magnetism, whenever the neophyte healer pulls back the disease of the to-be healed, the healer becomes more diseased than the patient. This is because he has tried to heal without learning how to transform his own mind into consciousness. Only consciousness may cure the lower mind. There is an ancient yogic saying, "Let your ego-mind stand aside and let the universal life-force energy do the healing." Only the higher yogis can do this because they are in a state of *unmani avasta* meaning an enlightened state of no-mind awareness.

A healer has to heal a patient and yet has to protect his own psychic integrity. How may this be done? Every time the healer heals, there is a resonant frequency. The healer's mind enters the mind and the body of the to-be healed and when it withdraws, it comes out with all the slush and disease and the negativity, which the healer absorbs into himself.

The healing processes cannot be done unless one masters the skills of the mind. One of the greatest healers of all times was Bhagwan Patanjali and he never spoke of healing. The best healing that can be done is to suffer your *karma*, go through it once and for all and be done with it. If you heal now, your *karma* will come back again. You cannot heal *karma*—you go through it or, due to your exceptional evolution, your Master takes it upon himself.

The Transformative Alchemy

Now I am speaking here of an esoteric psychology about which I have had experience. So I am not going to rely on referring to any books, but I am going to speak of my experience with *shaktipat* transmissions, so this is a very spiritual and intimate *goshti* (spiritual chat).

First, man's disease was primarily physical. We overcame it. The next prevailing disease was emotional and we are currently overcoming that by therapy. The future disease will be or rather is mental—of the mind. And that's exactly what has to be taken out of you. I have to forewarn you that the mind is used and overused. When the mind is overused, it is abused, and if you do not transform the mind, you will be in a mess. So the mind has to be taken charge of. Not by trying, but by witnessing the witness of the mind, you must resolve it to a state of calm and obedience. If you do try to willfully force the mind to obey you, it will react more violently. It may be compared to the violent reaction of drinking some water with bacteria in it and you throw up. You vomit and you feel you are vomiting your insides out. So if you try to force the mind to stop, so violent will be the reaction, that it will make a rag doll out of you and throw you out the window.

When I start to work on healing and transformation, I work on the various bodies of the disciple. I'm speaking about the spiritual bodies and the esoteric psychology of these bodies. I begin by working on the passion body, which is known as *Karma Sharir*, the body of passions, of raw emotions located at the navel center. Then on his body of emotions, which is centered in the solar heart of love which interpenetrates and envelops the passion body. And then I work on Divine Consciousness in the third eye which interpenetrates and envelopes both the passionate and the emotional body of love.

When I touch each center with divine energy of the Holy Spirit, one will feel there a vibration, heat, and light. Everybody may not feel the vibration, heat and light. They may feel only light and vibration, or only heat and sound, or see only light. This will depend on the degree of sensitivity of the individual or the degree to which one's subconscious mind is opened to the divine transmission, the *shaktipat* empowerment.

If someone is totally open in his physical and conscious mind and partially shut in his or her subconscious mind then he or she will not receive everything. If someone is totally open in the conscious mind and at the subconscious level, then he or she will receive the triple divine quality of light, vibration, and sound accompanied by heat.

The *Satguru* envelopes the disciple in an aura and then transmits the *shaktipat* transmission of *Kundalini* energy in the navel center. This is the way it is done. There is a connection and the Master gives the disciple a sensation of the triple divine quality, that is, the Divine light, vibration and sound, with his *Kundalini* energy when giving the *shaktipat*. This is accompanied by heat.

Now Divine light, vibration and sound are the alchemy that transmutes the base ore of passions into emotions. This body energy of desire is transformed and transmuted into the body of pure emotion and taken to the heart center. Now those desires, which can be transformed into emotions are taken up to the heart center to merge with the higher emotions. But those that cannot be transformed are kept there by the *nadis*, the psychic tubes of venous energy. The *Satguru* pulls into himself the emotional negativity and all the poisonous toxins from the disciple's body, drinks the poison and transforms it later into higher emotions and love.

Then he goes to the heart center, the *ananda kanda*, which is the center of emotions. There again he works the divine alchemy on the solar heart. Within the solar heart there is a lotus center, called the *anahat chakra*, a twelve-petal golden lotus. Within the *anahat chakra*, and a little lower, is an eight-petal rose lotus, which is called the *ananda kanda*, the seat of Joy. In the golden lotus of the heart *chakra*, the Guru transforms emotions into love, the highest quality of emotions. He also gives a technique whereby one may practice and progress into one's own divine loving nature.

Then the master goes on to work in the third eye center, the *agya chakra*, where he transforms love to divine consciousness by techniques like the *yoni mudra*, and by giving his disciple the experience of *shivapat*, his yogic Consciousness. If I bring about my *shivapat* happening of still-mind state, and everybody is tuned into it, they will all get my unified consciousness of thoughtless awareness. When Masters sit before you, you may see their bodies disintegrate and fall apart, change shape and become liquid and become fire and become light. Many of my disciples have seen this with their own eyes during *shivapat*. This is an encouragement for all who behold the Master's transformation into subtler dimensions to move on and to evolve to a higher sense of being, not by outward grasp, but by inward flow. The out-of-body experience and its psychedelic-like effects may also be given to many people at the same time.

The goal is the roots and wings of a well-balanced person with his practical feet well rooted in the earth and his work while his supra-conscious wings fly high in *samadhi*. Man tries to imitate the birds externally but knows not that he himself has a greater power and a greater ability to fly, but not with his physical body. Don't be stuck on that. Don't get hooked onto it—that one must, in his physical body, fly. No. Interpenetrating and yet enveloping the physical body, there are the subtler bodies that can be released and can take flight. It can go to any place within the speed of light. This is man's capacity. This is the truth. People have done it and people are doing it.

CHAPTER 12

SUPRA CONSCIOUS STATES OF YOGA
The Alpha & Omega of Yoga is Self-Realization

Yoga is the ascent of one's Consciousness through ever more refined and ever more expanded spheres of mind to get to the God-essence lying at the core of one's own Being. Yoga is brought about and made successful by *abhyasa* and *vairagya*. The meaning of *abhyasa* is to move towards the goal with intensity—towards God, unruffled by emotion or outward distractions. *Vairagya* means non-attachment to the objects of the five senses. *Abhyasa* assists in the cultivation of *vairagya*.

On our pilgrimage to the divine through the supra-conscious states of Yoga, three factors are necessary for the successful journey. They are perseverance in Yoga, unruffled emotions and reverence for the practice. The brave yogi has embarked on a journey to the holy of holies, from which the sacredness of all pilgrimages is derived. In the high stages of Yoga, he treads the sacred ground of ever more refined spheres of consciousness, as he nears the temple of *samadhi* in which his deity is enshrined.

When we consider the state of *samadhi*, we must be aware of the fact that this "technique" is not only the higher form of Yoga but its very essence. The great Rishi Vyasa has stated, *"Yogah Samadhi"* —*Yoga is Samadhi*.

It becomes necessary to point out that there is a widely prevalent misconception in the West regarding the nature and purpose of Yoga. A person practicing *asanas* and physical postures to improve his health says he is practicing Yoga. It's true that people in innocent ignorance vulgarize Yoga. Since a practice of *asanas* and postures does not constitute the real practice of Yoga - an individual can master all the 840,000 *asanas* without having a ghost of an idea about the true Yoga. On the other hand, a yogi can practice the real Yoga of *samadhi* without doing any *asanas*. So the physical postures alone only qualify a student to say he practices *asanas* to prepare for Yoga.

Another widely held and prevalent misconception is the one about diet. It is true that we need pure and *sattvic* food to put the body into the required state of harmony for the practice of Yoga. Many people in India habitually live on a diet of rice, curds, vegetables and fruits, which are *sattvic*, so they might as well claim they are practicing Yoga through diet. This is not the complete picture. The proper understanding is that both postures and diet are supportive to attaining the supra-conscious states of Yoga, but do not in themselves constitute Yoga proper.

There is no doubt that *samadhis* (the supra-conscious states) are the essential pathways of peace and Yoga. They must be practiced with proper preparation and prolonged graduated training. There are a number of scientific techniques integrated into a systematic but elastic course of discipline. The serious student of Yoga should follow these time-tried methods with the determination to reach the goal no matter what the temporary difficulties encountered or the number of lives it may take to reach the final *moksha*. This is not to be confused with easy shortcut methods given by pseudo-Yoga teachers to attract huge masses of followers.

One of the most critical factors to be cautious of is to know the difference between the psychic state of trance and the enlightened state of *samadhi*. When a person emerges from the supra-conscious state of *Samadhi*, he is aglow with the wisdom of the gods, for he has touched the feet of the Lord, his *Paramatma*. When a person comes out of a trance induced by other methods he goes to the lower mental and astral planes, without receiving any knowledge - he is the same as he was before. In the nineteenth and twentieth centuries, when Yoga was introduced to the west, for lack of a better word, trance was used to explain *samadhi*. This led to a lot of confusion because all psychics in trance were happy to be co-equal to the Buddha. But later they were put in their proper places when their psychic state of trance was explained to them.

The Ashtanga Yoga of Patanjali

Everything comes to him who makes the utmost effort under the circumstances in which he has been placed, as *Reeth*, the underlying order of the unfolding universe brings to each individual. The external Yoga consists of *yama, niyama, asana, pranayama*, and *pratyahara*. Their function is to prepare the *yogi* for the internal *Yoga*, which deals with the mind and comprises three techniques *dharana, dhyana,* and *samadhi*.

1. *Yama*: deals with the elimination of lower desires and emotions. It exercises moral precepts such as non-violence, truthfulness, non-stealing, sexual abstinence, and non-attachment.

2. *Niyama*: provides the disciplined ground for Yoga. This builds character so essential for success in Yoga. The five virtues to be practiced are purity in body and thought, contentment, self-discipline (*tapas*), meditation (*swadhaya*) and surrender to one's Divine Indweller (*Ishwar Pranidhana*).

3. *Asana* (postural integration): eliminates disturbances to the mind caused by the body, by making the body a fit instrument to progress in Yoga.

4. *Pranayama* (life-force control): eliminates disturbances caused by the three humors in the *pranic* body, gives control of the currents of *prana* and *apana*, which automatically makes *pratyahara* happen.

5. *Pratyahara* (reversal of the life-force energy *prana*): Eliminates disturbances coming through the sense organs by introverting the *prana* in the spine which gets magnetized, cutting off the five sense telephones from external objects. A yogi in *pratyahara* is like a tortoise retracting its limbs into its shell *(Goraksha Paddati* 2.24).

6. *Dharana* (concentration): With the mind left alone undisturbed by outer distractions yet filled with desires and their stored impressions. It becomes necessary to eliminate them by concentration. The merger of concentration into meditation is as natural as the flower becoming the fruit.

7. *Dhyana* (meditation): As the conscious state of meditation becomes more and more refined, the desires and their stored impressions (*samskaras*) weaken and lose their hold. Then a flowing state of awareness dawns that gradually transforms into expanded states of *samadhi*.

8. *Samadhi* (supra-conscious states of awareness): They are broadly *samprajnata samadhi, asamprajnata samadhi, nirbija samadhi,* and *dharma megha samadhi*. Then the yogi's consciousness expands into the truth of his infinite Self called *Niranjana Nirvana, Brahma Nirvana* or *Kaivalya*.

The processes of *dharana, dhyana,* and *samadhi* flow and flower into one another. These are three continuing stages of the same mental process. They differ in degree and not in kind. The fusion of the three phases in their totality is called *samyama* (becoming the object.) When a yogi takes an object in manifestation and applies *dharana, dhyana,* and *samadhi* to it until the reality hidden within the object is revealed, he is said to have performed *samyama*.

The Kriya Yoga of Babaji:

The prana apana yagya is the sacred fire ceremony of the yogi whereby he offers the oblations of *pranic* breath into *apanic* breath and vice-versa, to equalize the two life currents and enter the state of *kevali samadhi*.

There never has been nor will be a time when man's own nature shall cease to demand his best and foremost attention. The science of Yoga commends itself to the foremost minds of east and west. So vital is this inner science for the evolution of human consciousness that beside it, the greatest of human achievements pale into insignificance.

The science of *Kriya Yoga pranayam* offers the inhaled *pranic* breath into the exhaled *apanic* breath and vice versa. By this process the yogi neutralizes the two life currents of *prana* and *apana*. This results in the arresting of decay and growth in the body. This is done by rejuvenating the blood and body cells with life energy (*prana*) that has been distilled from the breath and moved into the spine and the brain. The *Kriya* yogi arrests all bodily decay, thereby quieting the breath and heart. This renders the purifying actions of the breath and heart unnecessary as they gradually slow down through persevering practice.

The *Bhagavad Gita* mentions this science of *Kriya Yoga* in chapter 4 verse 29. The *Kriya Yoga pranayama* called the *prana-apanic* fire rite by the yogis, teaches man to untie the cord of breath that binds our soul to the bodily cage. The soul is then released to fly and expand into the super-conscious skies of omnipresent spirit and come back at will into the little body cage. No flight of fancy is this, but a true experiencing of divine bliss.

Pranayama is derived from its Sanskrit roots, *prana* (life) and *ayama* (control). So *pranayama* is therefore life-force control and not breath control. In the larger sense, the whole world is filled with the

217

universal life-force energy called *prana*. Everything is a differentiation of the modes of expression of this universal force. Therefore, universal *prana* is *Para-Prakriti* (pure Nature). This eminent energy is derived from the infinite spirit and permeates and sustains the universe.

Individual *prana* is an intelligent force but has no consciousness in the empirical or transcendental sense. The Soul is the conscious unit and *prana* is its basis. The consciousness through mind-ego dictates terms and *prana* follows the dictate. Neither grossly material nor purely spiritual, *prana* borrows from the soul its power of activating the body.

There are two main life-currents in the body. One is that of *prana* which flows from the coccyx to the point between the eyebrows. The nature of this life current is soothing. It introverts the devotee's attention during sleep and the wakeful state, and in meditation unites the soul with the spirit in the third ventricle of the brain called the *shiva netra* or third eye.

The other main current is that of *apana* which flows from the third eye to the coccyx. This downward flowing extroverted current distributes itself through the coccyx center to the motor-sensory nerves. It keeps man's consciousness delusively tied to the body. The *apana* current is restless and engrosses man in sensory experiences.

"Greater is the yogi than body-disciplining ascetics, greater even than the followers of wisdom's path. Greater than the path of action. Be thou Arjuna a yogi!" (*Bhagavad Gita*, chapter 6 verse 46)

Kriya Yoga pranayama arrests bodily decay connected with *apana*, manifesting in the exhaling breath, by fresh inhalations of life-force (*prana*) distilled from the inhaling breath. This *prana* enables the devotee to do away with the illusion of decay and mutation. He then realizes that his body is made of "lifetrons" of congealed light. The body of the *Kriya* yogi is recharged with extra energy distilled from the breath and energized by the tremendous dynamo of energy generated in the spine. The decay of body tissues decreases. This ultimately makes unnecessary the blood cleansing functions of the heart. The heart pump becomes quiet owing to the non-pumping of venous blood and exhalation and inhalation of breath are evened out. The life energy unites in the currents in the spine. The light of pure *prana* scintillates from the six *chakras* to all the bodily cells keeping them in a spiritually magnetized condition.

Kriya Yoga is referred to obliquely in Yoga treatises as *kevali pranayama* or *kevali kumbhaka*. This is the true *pranayama* that has transcended the necessity for inhalation (*puraka*) and exhalation (*rechaka*); breath is transmuted into inner life-force currents under the complete control of the mind. When the breath stops effortlessly without either *rechaka* or *puraka*—that is *kevali kumbaka* (*Hatha Yoga Pradipika* II-73).

Of the various stages of *pranayama* (such as breathlessness), *kevali* is extolled by adept *yogis* as the best or highest (remember that *Kriya Yoga* is not breath control but life-force control). When one gets to the advanced state of *Shiva Shakti Kriya*, the breath ceases. Duly the cool ascending *pranic* current and warm descending *apanic* current are felt flowing in the *sushumna nadi* (spinal cord). This is an *avasta* (state) of *kevali kumbaka*.

Kriya is a process of converting breath into life-force and realizing the body as light. By the perfect performance of *Kriya* 1,728 times in one posture (that is, at one time) and by practicing a total of 20,736 *kriyas* a devotee can reach a state of *samadhi* (God contact). But *Kriya* cannot be practiced so many times by a beginner. When the body and mind of the yogi are prepared to accommodate the high voltage of so much *Kriya Yoga*, his Guru will advise him that he is ready for the experience of *samadhi*. If the *kriyas* are broken into several sittings, there is no harm. It will just take longer.

The *Gita* advises us to practice *pranayama* (life-force control) to enable us to realize that we are not made of flesh, but of life-force condensed from the thought of God!

The Omkar Kriya (Pranava)

The *Om kriya* practiced intensively in *Kriya Yoga* is also called the *pranava* (which means "the First Boat"). The "First Boat" of *Om* vibrations is built up by the ceaseless and devoted chanting of the sacred syllable in order to cross the "ocean of life" (*samsara*). These highly charged vibrations of *Om* form the desired protective vortex that makes you well-shielded against the storms and hazards of life and takes you to the haven of Self-Realization. I use the word vortex because it is the most potent junction between mind and spirit.

I have explained that *Om* is the seed vibration of the Divine Name. This light sound vibration of *Om* is the primeval atom from whence our three-dimensional universe began. It is advisable to begin all meditative practices with the *Om* technique and end the *Kriya Yoga* with *Om* meditation. This preserves the sacred spiritual power and love generated during daily practices.

The sacred sound vibration of *Om* is at first chanted loudly and then the meditation is more to listen to the sound in the right ear. By constant practice the inner sound gains velocity to express itself as light in the third eye (the space between and behind the eyebrows) as the sacred *Om* is a light-sound vibration. The sound is bound to express light in our consciousness, and burn past evil *karma*.

This technique of *Om* combined with the *yoni mudra* is a very effective and powerful meditation for rapid spiritual growth. This is one of the finest pathways for the evolution of spiritual consciousness.

Kundalini Kriya Yoga

Kundalini is the electro-magnetic *pranic* energy which means "coiled spiral" and stems from an earlier root *kunda* meaning "fire pit". It is coiled three and a half times around the base of the spine. *Kundalini* is represented by a cobra snake and can move a *yogi* from static state to kinetic activation in a split second. The *kundalini* is intensified spiritual *prana*. If the *pranic* energy is the atomic bomb, the voltage of the *kundalini* benefits the guided yogi like the hydrogen bomb. This awakened *kundalini* is one of the most potent boosts for any spiritual practitioner.

The *kundalini shakti* (force) is activated and awakened during the *Kriya Yoga pranayama*, which I call the *kundalini* breath. It is hidden and latent within all human beings in their nervous system. When the *Kriya Yoga pranayama* is performed as per the *Satguru's* guidance, the *pranic* life-force in your spinal cord (*sushumna*) builds up to generate a great spiritual magnetism and voltage. By the ceaseless movement of the *Kriya* life-force breath, one's *prana*, breath, vital fluid and mind become one to form the evolutionary life-force energy called *kundalini*.

According to the *Nath* tradition in India, the *Kundalini* is revered as the Divine virgin, the consort, the divorcee and the widow, all in One. She is the universal life-force of sustenance and evolution. At the base of the spine, the sleeping beauty Shakti awaits her Lord Charming Shiva's kiss of Consciousness, which releases her to ascend up the spine and unite with him in holy communion at the thousand-petalled-lotus. *Shakti - Kundalini* is the bride Cinderella, the "lady of the cinders" whom when fanned by the alchemical fire of *Shiva-shakti Kriya* ignites as *kundalini*, blazing up the chimney of the spinal *sushumna* to unite with immortal Lord Shiva in the crown *chakra*.

Yoni Mudra : Penetrating the Stargate

The *Yoni Mudra* (*Shanmuki Mudra*) is a light and sound technique of **Prathyahara**. Shiva Goraksha Babaji says, "As a tortoise withdraws its limbs into its shell so also by Yoni Mudra a Yogi withdraws his five senses into his consciousness." (*Goraksha Paddati 2.24*) It is essentially a technique to master the art of the withdrawal of mind and *prana* (life-force energy) from the objects perceived through the five senses. With *kechari mudra* it leads one right up through the states of concentration and meditation, so that the yogi penetrates the "stargate" of the third eye to enter into omnipresent bliss of *samadhi*.

Yoni means "womb" or "source". *Mudra* means "seal". It is also called the *jyoti mudra*, meaning "inner starlight seal". A third name is *shanmuki mudra*, because *shan* means "six" and *mukhi* means "orifice" or "mouth", and in this technique, the seven orifices are sealed so that the inner star of the Soul can be perceived, passing through which the Conscious Seer experiences Cosmic Consciousness.

By *yoni mudra* your mind is brought to a state of relaxed absorption, whereby *pratyahara* (sense withdrawal) ensues. This state of sense withdrawal occurs because of the pressure of the fingers upon specific nerves and acupressure points.

There are also physical benefits of *yoni mudra* because it stimulates the vagus nerves through pressure on the ear canals with the thumbs. The stimulation of these nerves brings about a dominance of the parasympathetic nervous system lowering the metabolic threshold; consequently bringing about the control of involuntary functions. The heart rate is reduced and the heart rested. Blood pressure is brought to a calmer state. The digestive system is toned and improved. The nervous system is rejuvenated, which brings about an equipoise of body and mind. One needs to be initiated into the sacred *Kriya* techniques. I have only given a brief synopsis of *Omkar, Kriya Pranayam*, and *Yoni Mudra*; the sequence of the preliminary techniques is given on the next page.

Sequence of Kriya Techniques

1. Omkar Kriya: The Birthing 'Hum' of Creation introduces one to his Divine Indweller.

2. Shiva Shakti Kriya: This yoga is the Kundalini Energy in motion. It is the raison d'être of Kundalini Yoga. It deals with the highest evolution of humanity and is rightly called the 'Science of all Sciences'.

3. Nabhi Kriya: Gaining equanimity of mind and thereby centering into yourself.

4. Mahamudra: The purpose is to open the flow of life energy in the spine by realignment. Integration of the physical, emotional and mental bodies is achieved by specific postures, Pranic Breathing, and Light Visualisations.

5. Khechari Mudra: An Inner Astral Flight and Rejuvenating technique which arrests the aging process.

6. Jyoti Mudra: Light and Sound Meditation whereby the 'Hamsa Soul' is seen as the 'Life Star of Light'.

7. Paravasta (Living in the **Enlightened Now**): This is Paravasta, the state of Being in the Present Awareness.

And we end with the following virtues, which are essential ingredients of the science of Kriya Yoga to be developed by the yogi: *Tapah* is the *Kriya* of self-directed austerities to strengthen your will, which looses the grip of your ego on creature comforts. It tempers and fine tunes your body and mind to enter deeper states of Yoga. *Swadhaya* is the Kriya of self-directed study brings about a deeper understanding of your true Self (the Concious-Seer) as opposed to your apparent self (the body-mind) by developing your *vivek* (discernment). *Ishvar Pranidhan*: individual yogic effort is important in the sojourn to Realization, but it is unconditional love for the *Sat-Guru* who represents grace which opens the portals of your heart to Self-Realization.

YOGA IS SAMADHI

SABIJA SAMADHI:
THE CONSCIOUS ECSTASY OF YOGA

In this section I am addressing you directly as I explain the journey of the *Hamsa* swan, your soul consciousness. *Samadhi* is described as an expanded state of consciousness which gives you the knowledge of the universe, God and man. However this may only be experienced when you, the Conscious Seer, transcend the senses, mind and intellect. When the mind becomes calmer by *Kriya* Meditation, you gradually aware yourself into the Divine Truth, Consciousness and Bliss. This is your own true Self.

There are two kinds of *samadhi* called *samprajnata* or *sabija* (with seed) and *asamprajnata* or *nirbija* (seedless.) The *sabija samadhi* penetrates the essence of Divine mind and the *nirbija samadhi* penetrates the essence of Divine Consciousness. The *sabija* includes the four states of *samprajnata samadhi*.

Sabija samadhi is that variety of *samadhi* in which the yogi has a definite object on which *samayama* is performed and its reality revealed as already shown. The yogic state of *samadhi* with seed is concerned with and utilized in unraveling the secrets of all kinds of things in the realm of mind and manifestation. In *sabija samadhi*, the yogi by *samayama* (becoming the object) finds the innermost secrets of any natural phenomenon and becomes a *Siddha* by accomplishing the *siddhis*. Any person with the sufficient will and perseverance is able to unlock the secrets of mother nature.

From age to age, great masters and scientists of their respective vocations have contributed to the progress of civilization and the evolution of the human race by discovering and disseminating to the people such knowledge gained by means of *samayama* and otherwise. The sun of spiritual consciousness shines eternally in the heart of every human being and he can discover any secret in the realm of nature if he has mastery of the technique. It is advisable to get guidance from a *Sat-Guru* who himself has tread the path. *Sabija samadhi* is further divided into conscious, supra-conscious ecstasies as given below. *nirbija samadhi* culminates in the *dharma mega samadhi*, the supreme conscious ecstasy.

SAMPRAJNATA SAMADHI:
THE CONSCIOUS ECSTASIES OF KRIYA YOGA

In classical Yoga, a series of ecstatic experiences are given which have an objective, mental content (*pratyaya*) with which consciousness (*chaitanya*) becomes identified, and which is related with supra-consciousness (*prajna*). As per *The Yoga Sutras* of *Patanjali*, there are four types of *samadhi* (subdivisions of the *samprajnata samadhi*), which corresponds to the *savikalpa samadhi* of the *Vedanta*. In any case both *samprajnata* and *asamprajnata samadhi* come under the category of *sabija samadhi* and are used alternatively to get to the stage of *nirbija samadhi*. The first is *samadhi* with seed as there is a definite object on which *samayama* is performed and the essence of the object realized when concentration, meditation and *samadhi* become one. When the three components of the mental process referred to as knower, knowing and known become fused into one homogeneous state of consciousness, then *samayama* is achieved and *samadhi* experienced. In this light the inner reality of the object (*siddhi*) is realized.

The Four Avastas (states) of Samprajnata Samadhi are:

a) *Vitarka Samadhi* is the first Yoga of focused awareness by analytical introspection on the gross physical form of your object of meditation. Your consciousness becomes intimately connected with the object on the level of its gross physical form. With your focus becoming steadier, your center of consciousness enters the next *samadhi*, understanding the deeper substratum of the object that underlies its outer physical form. Then your conscious awareness flows into the next *Samadhi Yoga*.

b) *Vichara Samadhi* is the second Yoga of reflective contemplation. This stage is known by a lessening of thoughts and a more powerfully centered absorption of the gross physical form of the object of meditation. As you move along this path of *samadhi* you experience a joyous wonder as your consciousness merges into and becomes one with the object on a deeper level of its physical form. Here consciousness exhausts the mind's thought process by virtue of its Being. Consequently your mind stills more and more, as you, the Conscious Seer, effortlessly expand into the third dimension.

c) *Ananda Samadhi* the third Yoga of Divine bliss and love. This state is characterized by a further stilling of the mental processes and a passive (non-volitional) mind. Your consciousness however, transcends its awareness of the gross physical form of the object of its meditation. It awares itself into the vast ocean of Consciousness, love and bliss. This is the subtle underlying support of the gross physical form of the universe. Here you will experience your self as freely floating in a vast limitless ocean of bliss and unconditional love. It is in this state of ecstasy that you will understand and be absolutely convinced that you are an integral part of this loving peaceful creative force called *Sat Chit Ananda* (existence, consciousness and bliss). As the mind becomes more transparent and stilled, your consciousness expands to express itself in the fourth dimension of *Samadhi Yoga*.

d) *Asmita Samadhi* is the fourth Yoga *of Sat Chit Ananda* (existence, consciousness, bliss). This is the unified field of Divine mind (the undifferentiated radiant ether of existence, consciousness and bliss.) An ultimate knowing occurs here that

226

"all of creation is me". Here you, the Conscious Seer, become aware that not only are you an integral part of, but you are *Sat Chit Ananda* in its entirety, as reflected through Divine mind. During this *samadhi* you enter into oneness with the primal ocean of non-dual conscious energy that later becomes the third dimension and has not yet divided itself into individual qualities (*gunas* – the subatomic particles.) In this state is realized the generic pool of all individualized consciousness. Here the realization dawns that "At the level of Consciousness Humanity is One."

Here in the *asmita samadhi* all fear of death is removed and supreme satisfaction is experienced where you could want nothing better, nothing more. This may be the reason why many yogis linger here for long and do not make the effort for the yet higher and inconceivable *asamprajnata samadhi*, the supra-conscious state of Yoga.

ASAMPRAJNATA SAMADHI:
THE SUPRA-CONSCIOUS ECSTASY OF KRIYA YOGA

This process of awaring leads the aspirant or yogi to the state of contentless consciousness; it is a unified state of consciousness with no mental content. The *Asamprajnata Yoga* has great Divine awareness. In this supra-conscious dimension, subject and object become one, leaving behind no thoughts or ideation. In *Vedantic* parlance this state or *avasta* is called *nirvikalpa samadhi*, the formless ecstasy.

Before the dawn of the *asamprajnata samadhi*, the supra-conscious ecstasy, the conscious ecstasy of *samprajnata* with its *chitta* or mind of mental ideation is already dissolved. All that is left is the residue of subconscious tendencies called *samskaras*. Initially the *asamprajnata samadhi* can be maintained by the yogi only for brief periods of time. This is because the memory of powerful subconscious desires (*samskaras*) pulls the yogi back to the *samprajnata* consciousness, a lower state of waking Consciousness ecstasy.

The *samskaras* (remembered experiences) then surface from the subconscious depths of the mind's lake to reassert themselves to become a hindrance to the yogi's spiritual ascent. Nevertheless, the brave soul, undaunted, persists in his practice. His periods of natural breathlessness by consciousness becomes increasingly longer, until the subconscious thought deposits in his memory banks are completely transformed to pure mindlessness. After this has happened the *asamprajnata* supra-consciousness state of *prajna* gradually transforms itself into the *nirbija samadhi* state. The experiencing of a long series of a repetitive seedless *nirbija samadhi* leads the yogi into the final *avasta* state called the *dharma megha samadhi*.

During this Yoga, you, as pure Consciousness, transcend the fourth dimension of *samadhi*, the unified field of the universe, and enter temporarily and frequently from Divine mind awareness into the realms of Divine Consciousness. We must know that this *samadhi* is more illumined than the previous four *samadhis*. Here, rather than consciousness perceiving the different stages of itself reflected on the surface of mind-stuff, it temporarily disconnects with the mind and enters into its own boundless Consciousness. Each time the "stargate" of the third-eye is penetrated, a paradigm shift occurs and the fourth dimension of the conscious ecstasy of mind awakens into the fifth supra-conscious ecstasy of Consciousness. It is out of this ineffable dimension of supra-consciousness that the third dimensional mind was born. This is perceived as time, space, and matter in the sphere of our universe of relativity.

In the fifth dimension of *samadhi*, the depth and experience of *Sat Chit Ananda* is far more profound than that experienced during the fourth stage of *samadhi*. No words can describe the completeness of this most sublime experience. But nevertheless, your consciousness not being established in *nirbija* (seedless *samadhi*) shuttles from the conscious to the supra-consciousness ecstasies, only to be pulled back to the conscious ecstasy by past life memory impressions (*samskaras*).

Then by a long series of alternating conscious and supra-conscious *yogic* ecstasies, the stored impressions embedded in the mind exhaust themselves. This enables your consciousness to permanently disconnect from the mind and expand your awareness into the supreme conscious ecstasy of Yoga—*nirbija samadhi*. Then you, the Conscious Seer, the supreme swan, have won your "Wings to Freedom."

We must understand that the state of *asamprajnata* or *nirvikalpa samadhi*, although temporarily devoid of the seeds of grosser desire, are still fettered by the subtler subconscious desires of past lives and hence must still come under the category of *sabija samadhi*, a *samadhi* with seed.

Methods Of Samadhi Whereby Karma Is Dissolved

There are basically four types of restrictions (*nirodhas*) in the classical Yoga system as detailed below. These methods help dissolve the *karmas* of past and present lives latent in the subconscious strata of your memory banks.

The Four Nirodhas
(Restrictions of thoughts and forms)

Vritti Nirodha (restriction of gross thoughts): The fluctuations of the mind or the thoughts determine the temperament of a person. These whirling thoughts are restricted and dissolved by meditation (*dhyana*) because if they are not, the subtle impressions of thought generate new mental thoughts. This restriction of thoughts by the breathless state of still mind leads you to the conscious ecstasy of *samprajnata*.

Pratyaya Nirodha (restriction of mental ideation): This ideation is a thought form and is subtler than thoughts. It can be resolved by you, during the practice of *samprajnata samadhi*. You must prevent the visual image and resolve it back to the mind impression from which it arose, thereby weakening the link between your consciousness and the mind.

Samskar Nirodha (restriction of the stored impressions): This occurs at the level of supra-conscious ecstasy called the *asamprajnata samadhi*. Remembered experiences bubble up from the depths of the mind's lake to occur at this level of *samadhi*. Their transformation is accomplished here by the mind stilling itself by undifferentiated thought waves of *Om* vibration, enabling you, the Conscious Seer, to identify with your vaster Self and further sever your identification with the still mind.

Sarva Nirodha (complete restriction): This coincides with the realization of the cloud of forms. When the *yogi* ceaselessly awares himself into the *asmamprajnata samadhi* states, the cloud of the sub-atomic tendencies (*gunas*) is dissolved. Here the *gunas* of inertia, activity and luminosity are overcome and transformed. Then having crossed the barrier of relativity, you enter the seedless *samadhi* of Cosmic Consciousness.

The Three Parinams
(Transmutations of Consciousness)

The three *parinams* means the three transmutations of your consciousness as you extricate yourself from the mind stuff called *chitta*. By the practice of *parinams*, your consciousness experiences a step-by-step evolutionary expansion of itself, as it passes through the grosser mental states to enter the subtler ones. Finally the mind exhausts itself and you, the Conscious Seer, express yourself as the supra-conscious Seer.

By transmutation is meant the movement of consciousness by yogic practice from the grosser through to the subtler layers of mind thereby evolving and expressing more and more of your divine Self. There is no change but an expansion in the essence of the conscious seer as the mind is exhausted of all its attachments and *samskaras* (stored mental impressions). Each time a transmutation practice is perfected, the Conscious Seer or Divine Indweller expresses more of its Divinity. When the last of the transmutations is perfected by total awareness, your consciousness is free and blossoms to express your absolute Divinity.

Nirodha Parinam

This is the transmutation of consciousness by restriction of the mind. Each time a thought wave, visual image or stored impression arises, you must overpower it and dissolve it back to its source. Such a repeated restriction or suppression of mental processes transforms and refines the mind. Simultaneously, you become more aware of yourself as expanded consciousness.

When the yogi in meditation repeatedly raises himself up and out of the mind's lake to identify himself with his supra-consciousness, he severs the *karmic* link between his Conscious Seer and the mind's remembered experience from which the thought arose.

So it is clear that when you ceaselessly raise your consciousness to identify yourself as supra-consciousness and consequently restrict the mental processes (*vrittis*), a transmutation of consciousness happens, which evolves you to enter into the next evolutionary Yoga called the *samadhi parinam*.

Samadhi Parinam

Samadhi here implies a conscious ecstasy of focused awareness. During the first three stages of *samprajnata samadhi* even the suppressive wave of the former transformation becomes successively weaker. The mind substance becomes transformed and refined by fleeting experiences of *samadhi*, which occur during the intervals between successive suppressing waves.

You, the Conscious Seer, by being in a focused state of conscious ecstasy, subdue the still mind to a deeper quiet. As a result your consciousness transmutes to express more of your divine Self. It is after perfecting this practice that you will realize yourself as an integral part of the infinite consciousness called *Sat Chit Ananda*.

Ekagrata Parinam

Ekagrata here implies a supra-conscious ecstacy of focused awareness. Here the fourth stage of *samadhi* occurs. As the mind lies absolutely still and quiet, your consciousness enters its Supra-Conscious ecstasy easily, as each wave image is identical to the one that just subsided. The mind stuff becomes transformed solely by one dominant wave experience of supra-consciousness made possible by the Conscious Seer being in total undivided absorption of its vaster Self.

The mind as still as a crystal lake, enables you in focused absorption, to penetrate the "stargate" center of your homogenous divine mind consequently evolving and expanding you, the Conscious Seer, into Cosmic Consciousness where you experience yourself not only as an integral part of, but the whole of *Sat Chit Ananda*. You realize yourself as the whole of Truth, Consciousness and Bliss.

NIRBIJA SAMADHI
THE SUPREME CONSCIOUS ECSTASY OF YOGA

Your consciousness, having permanently severed its ties with the mind, is now established in the sixth dimension of supreme conscious ecstasy. The ripples of thought in the mind's lake subside as the mind now lies subservient to Consciousness. Sensory thoughts, mental ideation and past memory impressions, having been transformed and zeroed by past *samadhis,* may no longer arise to pull you down. There remains no possibility that any latent seed impression could propel you back into the *karmic* cycle of birth and death. Thus only this sixth stage of *samadhi* is called *nirbija* (seedless.)

The fifth stage (*asamaprajnata*) is temporarily seedless where the consciousness shuttles from desire to desireless *samadhis;* but in the sixth dimension your consciousness permanently separates from the seed desires and stored impressions of the mind of the universe, which is the source of all *karma.*

After long practice comes the *nirbija* or seedless *samadhi,* which is the forerunner of the supreme Conscious Yoga of *dharma megha samadhi* (content-less Consciousness). These divine dimensions of *samadhi,* like the rainbow, blend one into the other. The yogi, by transforming himself from the cocoon, becomes the butterfly of freedom and Self-Realization.

The mind cleaves no more to your conscious Self. It lies subdued like a rippleless luminous lake of molten glass, absolutely still, and mirrors the splendor of your Soul Consciousness. Your consciousness not only identifies with your boundless Consciousness of God-essence, but becomes It. You, the Conscious Seer, now shine in the splendor of your own effulgent glory!

The *nirbija samadhi* will thus be seen as the culmination of *sabija samadhi* and not an independent method of Yoga. It is internal to *sabija* as the later is internal to *dhyana,* and that to *dharana,* and that to *pratyahara,* and so on so forth. *Nirbija samadhi* itself culminates into *dharma megha samadhi,* which is the ultimate *samadhi* preceding God-realization (*Brahma Nirvana*). This *samadhi* is called *nirbija* (without seed) because there is no object that has to be mentally split open by *samayama* in order to find the reality. The reality in this realization is God-essence itself.

To understand clearly what *nirbija samadhi* means we have to recall that all objects dealt with in *sabija samadhi* are in the realm of relativity and manifestation. The realities hidden within them are a part of the divine mind, which is the basis of manifestation. So in *sabija samadhi,* not only are our objects limited and present in the realm of mind, but in finding its corresponding reality we penetrate only up to the divine mind.

The divine mind however, is a differentiation of the Divine Consciousness, which illumines the divine mind. It is in this Divine Consciousness—the reality underlying our universe—that our *Purushas* are rooted as parts of the Divine Consciousness. If therefore we are to find the realities of our real selves, we must dive deep to penetrate beyond our divine mind into the realm of Divine Consciousness—to realize it as our own eternal Self!

PRATI PRASAVA
THE INVOLUTION OF CREATION

This means the counter flow and involution of the three *gunas* of *sattva, rajas* and *tamas* back into the transcendental matrix of the divine nature from where they were born. *Prasava* on the other hand is the streaming forth of the constituents which compose nature. When a yogi is about to win liberation there occurs a process of dissolution of those forms related to the microcosms of the soul about to be enlightened.

From the womb of lightless light called *Amba*, "the Great Deep", is the primeval atom of *Omkar* born, which explodes with the light-sound of *Om* to give birth to the sub-atomic particles of the three qualities of *sattva*, *rajas* and *tamas*. Everything in our universe is composed of vibrational combinations of the three qualities of *sattva*, *rajas* and *tamas*. Electrons represent the *sattva* of luminosity and harmony. Protons represent *rajas*, passion and activity. Neutrons represent the *tamas* of inertia, ignorance and dullness. These building blocks of nature coalesce to form the five elements of ether, air, fire, water and earth. The purpose of nature as universe is to provide the evolutionary growth for the Soul.

For a being on the threshold of final enlightenment, nature has completed her work and the triad of *gunas* (the electrons, protons and neutrons) which compose the subtle mind-stuff, recede back into her undifferentiated matrix. This withdrawal of *gunas* is only for the soul, which expands into the knowingness of its own ineffable state of *Kaivalya*, the Supreme Enlightenment.

Then for you, who has won his liberation, a counter-flow of the constituents of nature begins to happen. As the purpose of life is fulfilled for the yogi, he follows the ascent of his consciousness through gross levels of matter to its source until the physical universe dissolves into the unified field. But for others, its physical form continues to exist and to provide common experiences for them until they in time evolve and express their Divine Consciousness. The reversal of the elements and sub-atomic particles of nature happen.

Now *Om*, the Holy Spirit, is the birthing light of creation—the seed of the mind of nature and the matter of the universe. Before she resolves and zeroes into herself, the sweet nurse of the universe showers you with all her blessings and then disappears into her own transcendental matrix.

DHARMA MEGHA SAMADHI

This is called the *samadhi* of "The Cloud of Forms." A clear exposition of this state is important if you are to understand the states of enlightenment in their complete sense.

After your awareness has been purified during the fourth, fifth, and sixth stages of *samadhi*, if you continue to discern between your conscious Self and mind-self then the *Dharma Megha Samadhi* is closer. Even the *Sat Chit Ananda* (Truth, Consciousness, and Bliss), as reflected by the unified field of the universe, must be understood to be rarified Divine matter. As the yogi advances through a repetitive series of seedless *samadhis,* he goes beyond the sixth dimension, which lies on the other side of "The Cloud of Forms". But the *Dharma Megha Samadhi* is withheld until the last vestige of *karmic samskara* is worked out. A person can experience illumination or enlightened states of *samadhi* and yet have subtle *karmic* stored impressions of past lives unresolved.

When the yogi is continuously and firmly established in seedless *samadhi*, he is called the *Yogarudh* (unequivocally established in the highest state of Cosmic Consciousness). All his subtle *karmic samskaras* have been worked out. To be more specific, a *Siddha* entering the fifth degree dimension of enlightenment is not the recipient of the *Dharma Megha Samadhi*. But an *Avdhoot / Avatar* having crossed the seventh degree dimensions will be showered with the blessings of the *Dharma Megha*.

The supreme ecstasy of the Cloud of Forms is the sixth and seventh dimension of yogic consciousness. It is truly impossible to describe this ineffable experience or do justice to this state of exalted Truth. In this supreme conscious ecstasy not only is your consciousness permanently disconnected from the mind but the very mind is no more. It resolves back into its own state of *Laya* (zero).

So subtle and close is the transition from *Dharma Megha Samadhi* to *Kaivalya* that it is inexplicable. This *Dharma Megha Samadhi* is neither the *dharma* nor the *megha* (in the sense we understand the words), but the actual and factual happening of the reality of *Kaivalya*. This happening is the actual showering of the virtue of *Kaivalya* itself.

Before the yogi wins his final liberation called *Kaivalya*, the divine mind of Mother Nature appears between him and the finality. This lightless light of the Rings-Pass-Not still appears between the yogi and final liberation. This incomprehensible effulgence of light is beyond the cloud of *Omkar** (the birthing hum of Creation).

Then beyond the comprehension of both mortals and gods, the showering of the supreme virtue happens—no more to happen that happens or doesn't happen. The yogi enters the ineffable Absolute called *Kaivalya*!

KAIVALYA : PARAM SHIVA
THE NON-BEING ESSENTIALITY!

It is impossible to put to pen such an ineffable and lofty state of Truth. A humble endeavor is being made here. **He goes beyond the naked singularity. His mass is infinite. He experiences his Center Everywhere and Circumference Nowhere. The *Yogeshwar* is in *Brahma Nirvana*, The Be-ness About Whom Naught May Be Said!**

---

*Omkar is the sacred seed of light-sound (smaller than the nucleus of an atom.) It contains everything that is to become the third dimensional universe. At the beginning of each cycle of creation it explodes forth from the womb of the absolute Mother and becomes the universe of space time and matter. The light-sound *Om* is the sound of instant creation—it is Mother Nature herself who showers the blessings on the yogi before she resolves herself back into her own transcendental matrix.

CHAPTER 13

WAY OF THE WHITE SWAN
The Journey of the Soul

The journey of our Soul (the "White Swan") is the cycle of involution of human consciousness through mind into matter and its subsequent evolution from matter to mind, back to Self-Realization. The path of going forth is called *pravritti marg* where one's consciousness gets involved in the mind, the senses and the material world. Forgetting its true nature, it garners the experiences of life in its state of avid delusion, as it tastes the desires in this university of the material world. It is buffeted by these attractions and repulsions, after being involved in the best of life, and having tasted the joys and miseries thereof.

The inner-spirit of the "Soul Swan" pushes it towards its own evolution, called the *nivritti marg*, the inward path of return. This is the evolutionary path of renunciation and detachment from the pleasures of *samsara*. Here our Soul Consciousness, called the "White Swan," begins to withdraw itself from the grosser sheath of matter to the subtler spheres of mind. The "Soul Swan" has begun its inner yogic ascent through ever more refined and ever more expanded spheres of consciousness until it gets to the "Divine Indweller" which lies at the core of its own being. Then our consciousness expands beyond our own being to the boundless Godessence of the infinite reality.

The "Way of the White Swan" is the evolution of human consciousness. This is the most comprehensive enterprise ever undertaken by humanity, compared to which the greatest of human achievements pale into insignificance. This process is Yoga which commends itself to the foremost minds of east and west. In the human brain exists the lateral ventricles in the shape of a swan poised in flight, with its wings thrust forward and head pointing to the back as though flying back to the future, faster than light. When a *Hamsa Yogi*, through meditation and *pranayama*, activates the *kundalini* energy, these ventricles in the brain open up. The two petals in the *agya chakra*, corresponding to the pituitary gland, open first. The yogi, at this stage, experiences *Hamsa* Consciousness, being breathed by the Divine Indweller, the universal *prana*.

The *sushumna nadi* (astral-psychic channel) in the spinal cord is the highway through which the *Kundalini* energy travels and the evolution of consciousness takes place. *Kundalini* is the kinetic energy remaining after the completion of the universe. This force lies in potential form as light/sound vibrations coiled around the *swayambhu linga* in the *mooladhara chakra*. To avail of it for one's own evolution and realization is the birthright of every human soul. It may be awakened by yogic procedures: *shakti sancharan* and best by *unmani*, a no-mind state of absorption.

As the *Hamsanath Yogi* progresses in the *Hamsa* meditation, the third eye opens up in the *agya chakra* and he goes into the *savikalpa* consciousness. Then by further practice, he penetrates the star of the eye and expands to the *Paramhansanath Yogi's* state of *nirvikalpa* consciousness, dwelling in the cave of *Brahma*, the brain's third ventricle. His awareness evolves further, beyond the I-ness of humanity, to settle in the spaces of the lateral Swan-like ventricles of the brain, where he becomes the *Siddha Nath Yogi*. After this, the mighty *Hamsa* Soul wins its Wings to Freedom. The subtle fibers of the Corona Radiata light up with Divine Effulgence and he takes flight into Cosmic Consciousness as the *Avadhootnath Yogi*. He experiences the total Divinity of and beyond creation, gaining the ultimate knowledge of *Tat Tvam Asi*—"That Thou Art". The yogi then merges into *Niranjana*, the final *Nirvana*, having attained the enlightenment of *Buddha* and *Christ*, the *Avadhootnath* yogi returns to the world no more. If, under rare circumstances, he ever does, it will be the descent of divinity as the *Avatarnath Yogi*.

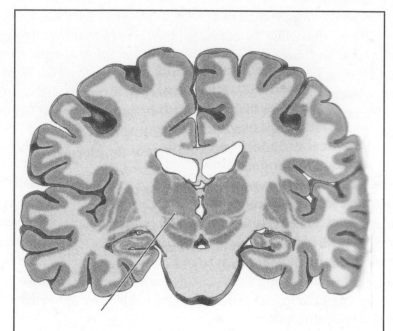

The Hamsa Swan, as I saw in meditation, symbolized as the lateral ventricles of the brain (shown above in white).

The Evolution of Human Consciousness

Entering the natural state, peering into the misty past of the *akashic* records of the ancient of days, I am blessed with the vision of the Sages of the Fire Mist and the mighty *Lakulish* of the Lilac Lagoons. Arising from the mystic waters of my consciousness, He holds in his hands the evolutionary lightning of life and death called *kundalini*. By his grace I see into the *akashic* records, the timeless evolution of human Consciousness. This is the *shramanic* knowledge of India predating the *vedas* and all world religions.

From time immemorial, Yoga, the sublime science of the Self, has come down to us. Those that hungered after the truth practiced and experienced for themselves that man is not a perishable body but an undying soul. His origin is Divine.

The end of physical evolution is the perfection of the mammalian form. The end of mental evolution is the perfection of the human mind. And the end of spiritual evolution is the full expression of one's Soul Consciousness of natural enlightenment.

From pre-historic mammalian man, with his mind enmeshed in the senses, we have gradually evolved to the human man with his mind centered in the intellect. Now we must follow the evolutionary process of Yoga whereby we may become Divine Beings of enlightenment by practicing these ways to enter the natural state.

The Furthering of Human Awareness by Yogic Initiation

The evolutionary process of Yoga whereby we may become Divine Beings is brought about by a series of initiations, which leads to the expansion of consciousness. This process is brought about by the definite intermediation of the Guru who acts in place of the Great Initiator of humanity, giving you a spiritual birth in his name. This furthering of human awareness gives the key to knowledge and opens up new centers of power so that the soul becomes more and more aware of itself, to become more serviceable to the world.

Man has seven *pranic chakras*, seven bodies which are composed of seven states of matter, each rarer than the previous one in density and corresponding to the matter of the seven heavens. There are seven layers of *kundalini shakti* used during the seven initiations in this world. Each *kundalini* initiation liberates the seven layers of consciousness to function in their respective bodies and their respective heavenly states. Any initiation beyond the seventh will take the individual soul out of the magneto-spiritual influence of this world and it can come back no more until the great world cycle is over.

There are seven great initiations which mark the stages of the spiritual progress of the path, each divided into four sub-stages, whereby the *Sat-Guru* and *Divya-Guru* take upon themselves the instruction and guardianship of the disciple. **Then under the guidance of a Master, this evolutionary path becomes simple and easy to practice. We must not be discouraged by the dizzying heights you have to climb, which we will climb because it is our birthright to do so. By the grace of the Sat-guru (Master), you will realize yourself flowering into the likeness of your ow divinity. So brave soul, be not disheartened, march on!**

First Level Initiation: *Hamsa-Sevak (Hamsa Dvij)*

Hamsa-Sevaks are those who have entered the stream of selfless service and work for the welfare of the human race, each according to his/her capacity. They are dedicated to serving humanity as their larger Self. They go where their Guru sends them - they want no more of the world except to be there as an element of service. They do what the Master wants them to do. *Hamsa Sevaks* are born anew. They are *Dvij*, and this is the first time they realize that they form a connection between humanity and Divinity by service to both.

The *Hamsa-Sevaks* are dedicated to the *Second Declaration of Human Rights for Earth Peace*:

To Serve Humanity as One's Larger Self by Earth Peace meditations every full moon, absorbing its peaceful rays within, and radiating the same to the world without.

Second Level Initiation: *Hamsacharya*

This is the next level of the expansion of one's Soul Consciousness. A *Hamsacharya* serves the human race to a greater extent by selflessly teaching sincere disciples the ways and means to realize themselves. He needs steadfastness and not to bow down or to turn back. Though everything seems against him at times, he must have courage in his convictions to work on, and know that all is working for his ultimate good.

It may appear unjust that when he is trying his best, the worst befalls him, and when he is living better than he ever did, all difficulties assail him. It seems quite unjust and hard that the noble cause he pursues should bring him such hardships. He must refuse in his mind to be disturbed, even by apparent injustice, for it is not injustice that he is reaping in this life, but justice and the fruits in this life of the seeds sown in his past lives (*karma*). If illness strikes him, he must think that much *karmic* debt is being paid. He is the stronger for it. When pain and anxiety assail him, he is paying the debt of sorrow, and his thought should be, "Never mind if my body is naked and shivering. I must not leave my soul naked and shivering."

The *Hamsacharya* is joyful in the midst of sorrow, hopeful in the midst of discouragement, and steadfast (*stitha-pradnya*) in the midst of difficulties. He is content and knows that the great ones and the law of *karma* are working for his salvation. The *Hamsacharya*, by sincere spiritual practice, may attain to liberation in this very life and return to earth but once more for the service of humanity in better circumstances.

Hamsacharyas are dedicated to the *Third Declaration of Human Rights for Earth Peace*:

Use the way of the peaceful breath that flows equally in all as a means for attaining world peace, thereby diffusing individual and international conflicts by the *Hamsa* way (*Gurunath Samadhi Yoga*). The journey of the Soul comprises the expansion of consciousness either through a series of Yogic initiations or by natural evolution, a much slower process.

Third Level Initiation: *Hamsanath Yogi* (*Hamsa Kriyacharya*)

Through the Guru's grace, the initiate enters into the no-mind stage or *sahaj samadhi*, experiencing the no-mind state of natural enlightenment.

The *Hamsanath Yogi* knows that he is united with the Divine. "*Ham*" is "I am" and "*Sa*" is "He." The *jiva* comes in as the sound of "*Sa*" and goes out with the sound of "*Ham*". The *Hamsanath* yogi, due to sincere spiritual meditation in this life, is able to cut the fetters of bondage and *karma* and get his first liberation. He no longer needs to return to earth. However, more often than not, he is directed to return to earth to be of greater service to humanity, so as to propel the Soul's journey into more glorious realms of Consciousness.

Each stage of a major initiation is divided into four sub-stages, and the *Hamsanath Yogi* must be well aware of this fact as he passes through them. All the levels of initiations require the yogi to pass through the four sub-stages, until the fifth level is reached. The requirements for evolution after the fifth level of *Siddha* are little known to man. The four sub-stages are:

Marga: The first stage of the level of initiation. *Marga* means the way in which the disciple is striving to cast off the fetters.

Phala: The second stage of the level of initiation. *Phala* means when the fruits or results of *sadhana* begin showing.

Avasta (Bhava): The third stage of the level of initiation. *Bhava* means consummation and he is a master of the state in which he belongs—he is fully established in the awareness of the state.

Gotrabhu: The fourth stage of the level of initiation. He is now ripe and fit to receive the next initiation.

At the third level of initiation, the inner fire must be awakened. It is here that the *kundalini* must be roused to function in the physical and astral body of the initiate, leading it from *chakra* to *chakra*. As *kundalini* awakens, it gives man power to leave the physical body at will, disengaging the astral from the physical, setting it free to serve humanity as one's larger Self in a vaster theater of operation. Many of the powers and *siddhis* are also developed in this stage.

A word of caution - it is here that the danger of being ensnared by the ego lies. Some saints and yogis due to their past karmas become world teachers with large followings of admiring disciples. At the third and fourth stage, they must resist the temptation to pretend to be more than what they are. Some of these souls because of excessive *kundalini* surge may hallucinate themselves into believing they are Avatars (divine incarnations of the Mother or the Kalki Avatar *etc.*). They bask in the praises showered upon them by deluded devotees who haven't a clue about what an Avatar is. The saint or philanthrophist in turn makes no effort to correct their mistaken identity. This situation is detrimental to both the saint and the devotees.

> *Hiss Kundalini sting ego mine*
> *With nectar poison so sublime*
> *Penetrating all my lotus shrines*
> *Making me to myself Divine*

The *kundalini* awakens not in a state of concentration but in a state of *dhyana*, which is often mispronounced as zen. Now there is no requirement for concentration. Concentration means the faculty of exclusive attention. When there is concentration and attention, there is a tension, there is a stretching, an effort. *Dhyana* is effortless and flowers into the *sahaja samadhi* state.

When the yogi goes into a state of *sahaja samadhi* (natural state of equilibrium), it is a state of Shiva, a state of Shiva-ness. When Shiva is there as the eternal Divine Consciousness, then the Shakti simultaneously awakens and arises to meet her Lord. *Kundalini*, awakens more through absorption, rather than effort. The purpose of its awakening involves other states of divine evolution with which humanity is not too familiar as yet.

There are two ways of awakening the *kundalini*:

The *Hatha Yoga* process of *shakti chalan mudra*, *kechari mudra* and practicing the *bandahs*, the *agnisara* movement of the abdomen, *shad chakra bhedan* (the bumping of the root *chakra*s), and through the *omkar kriyas*.

The *Raja Yoga* process of awakening the *kundalini* by doing or entering the *unmani* state of still-mind expanded awareness. It is so thoroughly, utterly simple, and naked truth, that it is difficult for a man, who is complicated with day-to-day thoughts, to be absorbed in this profoundly simple state called *sahaja samadhi*, the natural state. Therefore, if one practices it, it will take him twelve years to thoroughly de-complicate his mind. It would mean going into or melting into a state of awareness, bereft of any threads of *karma*, or thoughts. *Patanjali's Yoga Sutras*, the *Bhagvad Gita*, and the Philosophy of Gorakshanath, were not only the greatest expositions but those who gave these works were also the greatest givers of Truth the world has ever witnessed.

Babaji Gorakshanath has given us this truth of practicing the various ways and means of speeding up our spiritual progress. He is the great "Lakulish of the Lilac Lagoons". The lilac lagoons are the depths of our own Soul Consciousness. He holds in his hands the *lakulish*, which represents the thunderbolt club of evolutionary lightning, surpassing of life and death. Far beyond the reckoning of not only mortal man but even of the Gods, this Nameless One, this visible Invisible Savior of mankind, whose consciousness is spread throughout eternity, is called "The Lightning Standing Still", also called the "Great

Initiator". He is the Great Initiator of past, present, and future. This evolutionary lightning is called the *kundalini*.

The *Hamsanath Yogi* is dedicated to the *Fourth Declaration of Human Rights for Earth Peace*:

One's inalienable right lies in the furthering of the evolution of human Consciousness for earth peace, by exercising one's will to do good for making one another's lives on this planet a celebration through *Shiva-Shakti* and *mahamudra*.

Fourth Level Initiation: *Paramhamsa-nath Yogi*

Such a one has passed the fourth great initiation. In his waking consciousness, he can rise to live in *satya loka*, the *turiya avasta*. The consciousness of natural enlightenment is his while still aware of his physical body. He experiences waking consciousness on the *atmic* plane without loss of physical consciousness. The *Paramhamsa-nath*, at this stage throws off, dissolves the last five fetters:

Rup-raga: desire for life in form.
Arup-raga: desire for formless life.
Maana: pride. Its dissolution brings humility seeing and feeling all as one.
Uddhaka: restlessness. This transforms into *sthita-pradnya:* being nonchalant and not disturbed by anything. Knowing that peace is the most precious gift of God.
Avidya: the last film of ignorance, which hides the perfect Truth - It is the negative mind which covers the splendor of one's Soul.

All human lessons have been learned and such a one enters the consciousness of natural enlightenment at will for the salvation of humankind. This is a good work indeed—so essential for the further awakening of humanity. It is at this fourth stage of the *Paramhansa* that the fourth layer of *kundalini* is awakened and consolidated.

247

Kundalini has seven layers of consciousness. If all the seven layers of *kundalini* consciousness are awakened then the Soul totally disappears from the face of the earth. No man can awaken even his sixth layer of *kundalini* on this earth and live for a very long time. He must dissolve in Cosmic Consciousness. So we are talking about the Cosmic and individual *kundalini*. The Cosmic *Kundalini* you see for example, let us say, travels at 300,000 km/sec and individual *kundalini* travels at 30m/sec. You have got to bridge the gap between the Cosmic and the individual. Therefore, you need a transformer, a spiritual step-down system. This transformer is the *Satguru*, who speeds up the individual *kundalini* and heightens its rate, and lessens that of the Cosmic *Kundalini*, and then fuses them together to give the individual Soul an evolutionary boost. So the Soul-awareness takes a quantum leap, which could be too overpowering for the individual unless guided by the Guru. No more can be said on this subject unless in empowerments and initiations.

The Cosmic *Kundalini* is a totally different noumenon than the phenomenon of individual *kundalini*. As you attend more and more of the *Satguru's satsangs* or gatherings, you'll see the *Kundalini* at work—the radiance of *Satguru's* aura shown, the changing dimensions and the stillness experienced, are all the power of *Kundalini*. She is the serpent of the fathomless deep, *Aja Ek Pad* (The unborn standing on one foot). The *Ahirbudnya* (Serpent of the Fathomless Deep) the naked singularity, is Shiva fused with his Shakti, whom nobody can fathom; whom nobody can know intellectually in her ultimate seven-fold form. I am here speaking of the Cosmic *Kundalini*.

You can only be one—get absorbed and you will know all the past lives' experiences - reading the future and seeing the aura are the powers of *Kundalini* at work. She is called Shakti when united with Shiva. She is the "Mother of the Great Deep", *Amba*, also known as *Bal Tripura Sundari*, the "Cosmic Divine Beauty". Individually, she is the Divine bio-electric life-force which remains after the completion of the universe. She is tucked away in a bundle at the root *chakra* of every individual atom called the human being. It's our birthright to absorbingly beseech the awakening of the *kundalini* for the evolution of oneself, thereby to serve humanity as one's larger self. This is the sort of work I assist in. Of course, I cannot give you one trillionth of what she actually is, because man has never formulated words to describe what the *Kundalini* is. So, all our efforts are not telling us what she exactly is, they are just pointers to what we can do through practice—she is not exactly a subject of discussion but more of experience.

There are no instruments that are used, when I give the "Here Now Awareness" of Soul Consciousness, but everybody gets this experience simultaneously showing that at the level of Consciousness, humanity is One. We should investigate this by science but it needs more sophisticated tools. At present, we have only consciousness as a tool, one to another. It's a Guru-disciple relationship—my giving you my "Now Awareness" and you all experiencing it. This is what a sharing and caring of humanity is, and this is the way in which humanity is served as one's larger Self.

Fifth Level Initiation: *Siddhanath Yogi*

> *Then stiller than stillness itself*
> *With bated breath, I do behold*
> *My rising Self-Sun's nectar gold*
> *I dissolve in that mystery untold.*

The hierarchy of the *Siddha sangh* comprises the Guardian Wall of Humanity – this is the great *Nath Mandala*. The *Siddhanath Yogi* is dedicated to the *Fifth Declaration of Human Rights for World Peace*:

By virtue of being a world citizen it is one's inalienable right to attain the consciousness of natural enlightenment, leading to the realization that your expanded consciousness and humanity's consciousness is one. Further realize that humanity's consciousness as the world disciple is to be bridged with Divinity's Consciousness. The *Siddhanath Yogi* is the bridge, the *Tirthankar*, who not only builds the rainbow bridge between humanity and Divinity but sacrifices himself to be it!

As he lies across the chasm to form the bridge, human souls walk over him and pass through his aura of light to enter the realization of their Divinity. Such is the work of the *Nath Yogi* and *Nath Mandala* – to help evolve this World Disciple and bridge the gap between humanity and Divinity. The *Siddhanath yogi* gives directly the consciousness of natural enlightenment, the "Here Now" state of *sahaja samadhi*.

These great *Nath* Masters are one with the divine will and they are ever in the waking consciousness of Enlightenment. When out of the body, the *Siddhanath* rises to still higher states of Divine Consciousness. The experience is practically impossible to describe. Their service to humanity is the evolution of human consciousness leading to the realization that one's expanded Consciousness and humanity's consciousness are one. This is the fifth declaration of human rights for world peace which I have given. At all times, the *Siddha Sangh* generates spiritual power, sacrificing it and putting it to the service of humanity, using it for lifting the heavy burden of the world. Metaphorically, the *Siddha* is said to be Janus-faced, with one face absorbing the cosmic forces of other worlds and spheres of consciousness, transforming their potent effects into love and harmony. With the other face, transmitting to humanity the much-needed healing spiritual energy at a reduced and beneficial level, for their growth and evolution, thereby transforming them.

Sixth Level Initiation - *Avadhootnath Yogi*

The *Avadhootnath Yogi* means he who has completely cast off all limitations of body and mind. He is the Lord who has the power to grant boons, give protection, and bring about liberation. *Avadhootnath* is the Lord of ceaseless and persevering devotion, kept alive by the power of Yoga and sacrifice. The Seven Mighty Beings who have passed the sixth level of initiation have the power to focus within themselves the essence of all seven heavenly spheres of consciousness. These mighty *Avadhoots*, these seven *Naths* are the sun rays of the *Sapta Rishi*, the Seven Sages of our constellation called the Great Bear. Each is an overlord of one of the seven races, seven planets, and seven galaxies. You will see as the evolution of these souls proceeds that they expand to become one of the Sages of the Fire Mist, and one of the seven sages of the Great Bear, which are only their physical bodies. Their informing spirits are way beyond the comprehension of all mortal beings and even beyond Celestial Beings or *Devas*.

At this level of spiritual awakening stand two monumental Beings:
King Vikramaditya, descended from the solar dynasty of the house of Ikshavaku Ram and the world teacher Naga Arjun, descending from the house of the Krishna of the lunar dynasty.

Nath Vikramaditya (Chandragupta El Morya)
The Spiritual King

Vikramaditya in his former life was prince Balram, the brother of Lord Krishna and Naga-Arjun was the king Devapi. Vikaramaditya El Morya, an ancient Rajput prince, stands to serve humanity and the new and upcoming race with great strength and serenity. He teaches *Raja Yoga* and is connected with Lord Shiva's power, majesty, and spiritual glory.

People in whom the planet Mars and the sun star aspect are strong favorably bring about the quality of valor, courage and military genius as well as *Raja Yoga* practice. The King *Nath* Vikramaditya will evolve into the future *Manu Savarni* of the sixth root race. He is destined to be the future spiritual king of our world. Presently, he is at work in his astral body on the coast of California as well as the entire west coast—it is an India-California connection. I am of this Spiritual Master, doing the same spiritual work and of the same lineage.

Nath Naga-Arjun (*Devapi Koot-Humi*)
The Spiritual Teacher

He is to be the great world teacher and has to do with wisdom and *Jnana Yoga*. He is destined to succeed Maitreya, the present world teacher, and disciple of the supreme sage Parashar. It is prophesied in the *Kalki Purana*, and *Vishnu Purana*, that these two mighty Beings, Vikramaditya of the solar dynasty and Naga-Arjun of the Lunar dynasty, by their power of *tapas* and Yoga, are alive throughout the ages and shall establish a spiritual world beginning from the dawn of this millennium. Naga-Arjun's work is to do with the vibrations of the planet Mercury and the Moon. The Divine work of both these lofty Beings shall reach its zenith when the zodiac signs Leo-Aquarius shall be opposite to one another.

The *Avadhootnath Yogi* returns to the world no more. If under rare circumstances, he ever does, it will be the descent of Divinity in flesh in form as the *Avatarnath Yogi*. The *Avadhoot* is one who severs all worldly ties of attachment and is totally free from the *karma* of the world and of *devas* of the heavenly regions.

Seventh Level Initiation: *Avatarnath Yogi**

They are the true world teachers and divine rulers of all the humanities, past, present, and future. There are three mighty *Avatar-Nath Yogi*s who are at present governing our spiritual world:

1. The *Avatarnath* Vaivaswat Manu: The Spiritual King, son of Brahma Rishi Kashyapa, from whom descends Ikshavaku and then Rama Chandra (47th in descent from Ikshavaku) – the lineage is carried on to the Buddha and then from the house of Buddha

---

*For a comprehensive description of the *Avatar*, his role and work, as well as the forthcoming appearance of *Kalki Avatar*, refer to the next chapter on the *Avadhoot/Avatar* Doctrine.

descends Vikramaditya, and the solar dynasty of Suryavamshi, to which Yogiraj Siddhanath belongs.

2. The *Avatarnath* Maitreya: He whose ancestor is Varuna from whom descends his grandfather, the *Rishi* Vashishta who is the father of the *Rishi* Parashar. Next in descent from Parashar, is Maitreya who is our present world teacher, the wisdom of Vishnu. He will be coming in future as the Kalki Avatar. In esoteric circles, he is called *Sapta-Sapti*.

3. The *Avatarnath* Agastya: The son of the ancient *Rishi* Mitra, is the teacher of *Karma Yoga* and activity of Brahma; expansion, generation, and procreation of all species and especially the human race.

The *Avatar* Maitreya is the fifth secret Buddha and should in no way be confused with the *Purna Avatar* Krishna. This mistake is committed by many writers and needs clarification. Although the spirit of Krishna informs Maitreya, the latter is not of the spiritual evolution of Krishna, who is Divinity itself while Maitreya is Divinity in the making. Neophytes should be cautious of writing about the two or putting them at the same spiritual hierarchy.

The Work of the Avatarnath Yogi

During the whole period of a root race, our *Manu* Vaivaswat works out the details for the evolution of humanity affecting its *Atma,* that is, its Consciousness.

The *Jagat Guru Avatar*, world teacher Maitreya develops whatever spirituality is possible for humanity at that stage, affecting the level of *buddhi*, the intuition.

The Himalayan *Avatar* Agastya evolves *manas*, the mind, by *Karma Yoga*. He directs the minds of men through administration and different forms of culture and civilization, unfolding according to the cyclic plan. He affects the heart and head of an evolving humanity. From the Himalayas, at the behest of Mahadeva, he has come to make his presence felt in the Southern Hemisphere of the world.

Eighth Level: *Rudranath Yogi* — (*Shiva Kumar*)
The Sages of the Fire Mist

Four mighty Beings preside over the inner government of our galaxy and four pillars of the universe. Tradition whispers what the Gupta Vidya affirms. Reference is made in the Linga Purana of "the Inner Man," who only changes his body from time to time. He is ever the same, knowing neither rest nor *nirvana*, spurning the seven heavens and remaining constantly on earth for the salvation of humankind. Such are the seven virgin Sages of the Fire Mist, the *Shiva Kumars*. Four sacrifice themselves for the sins of the world and instruction of the ignorant, till the end of this world cycle (*manvantra*).

Though unseen they are ever present. People say of them, "he is dead, behold he is alive and under another form." Their bodies are composed of other-worldly lightless light. They are the undying, immortal ones, great beyond the reckoning of mortals. You should never speak their names in vain or before an uninitiated group of people, nor the names of the disciples of these great ones. The wise alone will understand.

These sacred four have been allegorized in the Linga Purana as the "Angels of the Face of God." The same holy text states that Shiva as the supreme Sage of the Fire Mist is born in each *kalpa* as sixteen virgin youths: four white, four red, four yellow and four brown. These are the sacred Sages in whom Shiva's spirit of Divine Wisdom and chaste asceticism incarnates. They are infused with his power. This connects with the epitaph of Babaji-Gorakshanath, "The Youth of Sixteen Summers."

These mighty Beings came to earth because our world was at the stage of evolution where we could receive the divine spark whereby the intellect or *buddhi* could be made possible. Without the guidance of these sages, the human mind would have plunged into a world of passion and animal nature. Because of these sages (the *Shiva Kumars*), the evolution of human consciousness was given a great impetus. They are the wondrous rulers of our spiritual government and dwell in Shvetdeep, a spiritual location beyond the Himalayas, in the aurora borealis of the northern lights. It is said that they brought the Sanskrit language to our planet from Venus and Sirius. A clearer understanding may be had of these beings by meditating on Shiva—so say the yogis.

The balance of the universe is rooted in reciprocity, and the foundation of the evolution of the world is sacrifice. Even at the high level of the Sages of the Fire Mist, the *Rudranath Yogis*, sacrifices are made to prepare great sages to undertake a greater work in the world.

Mystery Unveiled — The Solar Initiate

I am here telling you about one such sage called Surya. He is the guiding spirit behind our visible sun and his potential for evolution is great. In the Indian pantheon, he goes by various names, such as Narayana, Aditya, Kashyab. In one of the ancient scriptures, his spiritual status is extended right up to the God-essence, where the Surya sun is addressed as the seventh and highest spiritual sun. He is called Paramshiva in the *Aditya Hridayam mantra*.

There is a story of the *avatar* Ramchandra descended from Surya Narayana, the guiding spirit of our visible sun. He went into a state of sacrifice for the redemption of the sins of mankind. So *Surya*, the sun's highest spirit, descended into the nether regions and then into the world of mortals called *mrityu loka*, meaning "the land where death is inevitable." There the sun became *vikrant*, meaning shorn of celestial beams. This is an allegorical reference to the fourteen years of *Vanvasa* exile that the celestial Rama, underwent without his crown of splendor. In its stead, a crown of brambles was put on the sun's head, which symbolizes the sacrifice and hardships the Solar King underwent during his exile.

He also lost here his beloved *shakti*, his wife Sita, who was abducted by Ravana, the demon king of Atlantis Lanka. Then Rama the sun is made to roam the mortal world becoming a *karmasakshi*, a witness to their deeds. The reason why our solar gods and celestials roamed among the mortals was to take on their negative *karmas*—they would evolve humanity by infusing in its consciousness the fire of their Divine Spirit.

Having gone down to the haunts of men and suffered for them, and sacrificed for them, the *avatar* Ramchandra arose victorious and was installed as King of Ayodhya. He then became *Gabastiman*, full of radiant spiritual splendor. The sun initiate had successfully completed his trial and was ready to evolve to an even higher state to partake in a vaster order of cosmic work of Love and evolution.

Ninth Level: *Jaggannath Yogi* (Lord of the Universe)

> *Hold your silence stillness still*
> *For here your feet upon your head*
> *Your head humbled upon the floor*
> *The awe-filled mystery You! yourself*
> *Ask no more!*

The blank space above is in homage to this Nameless Being in an endeavor to express all the Is-ness of His Majesty, which cannot be expressed in callous limited words of the dumb human mind and tongue.

The space is dedicated to the Being About Whom Naught May Be Said. He plays with causation, space and time, as a child would play with soap bubbles, and if he were to smile in his innocence, he would shatter the world.

> *Who art Thou, I know Thee not*
> *And yet I am of Thee*
> *I cannot comprehend Thee Lord*
> *Thou Emperor of Divinity*
>
> *I sit and melt in Silence*
> *Of Thy Love Infinite*
> *Make me Thy Truth*
> *Make me Thy Love*
> *Eternal Lord of Light*

This initiation is not given by anyone to anyone, but is Self-taken. Shiva-Goraksha-Babaji is the deathless presence of eternity who keeps in His aura even the coming of the Kalki Avatar and all of the divine manifestations. It is not given to us to know what arrangement or spiritual impetus to humanity shall be given at the beginning of the new age, but it is said that a tremendous Being, a manifestation of *Shiva* himself shall incarnate at the end of the millennium, in one or many souls, and do as great a work on the spheres of the inner consciousness of humanity as the Kalki Avatar will do on the outer, at the junction of the Leo-Aquarius zodiac. Why this apparently premature spiritual boost is being given, only God knows.

Remember that humanity at large is not ready to awaken from its slothful, sweet slumber of delusion, illusion and error. Although a galvanic spiritual surge shall come from this great manifestation of Shiva, it will not damage the spiritual system of humanity, or its astral *chakras*, corpus callosum and brain system. The evolutionary surgery by this lofty Being is to prevent the extinction of humanity from the face of the earth, while spiritually enabling it to make the paradigm shift to a more enlightened state of awareness!

This immortal Being was never born. He is *aja* (deathless). He is the source of the *Nath* tradition of yogis, the great "Lakulish of the Lilac Lagoons," originating from the night of pre-history. The yogic tradition of the *Nath yogis* predates the *Vedas* and is *Shramanic* in its essence. At that time the ancient Babylonian, Egyptian, Chinese and Mayan civilizations existed only in their embryonic stages.

Great beyond the reckoning of mortals is the Spiritual King of our world who rises from the ocean of our innermost consciousness, the mighty "Lakulish of the Lilac Lagoon". Arising from the mystic depths, he holds in his hands the *Kundalini Shakti*, the lightning of immortality. He holds the mystery of life and death, directing the wholeness of the evolution* and dissolution of the world, not only of humanity but also of the *devas*, nature spirits, and all creatures connected with this world.

Babaji's consciousness is of such an extended nature that it comprehends the life and livingness on our globe, our galaxy, and our universe all at once. This nameless one is known as Shiva-Goraksha-Babaji, Ishvara Sanatana, and Mahavatar Babaji. He is the deathless Master of eternity, who has sacrificed himself for the redemption of existence for a whole universal cycle; a *Mahakalpa* of over 3 trillion, 110 billion, 400 million years; the life assigned to the whole of our Cosmic Creation—which is not even a wink of an eye in his Consciousness. He is *Maha-bhinishkaran*, "The Great Sacrifice," the highest "Be-ness", who explodes himself to enter the atoms of all sentient and non-sentient beings to evolve humanity and Creation to Divinity. **As the ceaseless sacrifice continues, this Divinity gives completely of Itself and yet remains complete.** This Divine enigma shall ever remain beyond the scope of our humanity and celestials to understand.

"Heaven and earth shall pass away, but I shall be with you to stay," says Babaji Gorakshanath.

---

*The evolution of the Soul depends not on time but on its past *prarabdhic* force of *sadhana* and present *purshartic* effort.

CHAPTER 14

THE AVADHOOT AVATAR DOCTRINE

In today's spiritual culture, the word *avatar* is being very loosely used without knowledge as to its true significance and what it really means. Anyone who can whip up a temporary hysteria is classified as an *"avatar"* by the masses who themselves haven't the slightest clue of what *"avatar"* means. In order to give people an understanding, it has become necessary to guide them and give a clear vision as to what an *avatar* actually is, the different types of *avatar*s, and what their work is.

The Divine Work and Advent of the Avatar

The word *avatar* is composed of two words, *ava* meaning to descend and *tara* meaning to save by bridging the gulf between humanity and Divinity. The Divine Consciousness descends to incarnate in the haunts of mortal beings to save their souls by ferrying them across the delusive ocean of *samsara* (the material world), into the haven of Self-Realization. This is the classic Indian thought coupled with the idea that the *avatar* deals with the spiritual evolution of human consciousness. Like the Biblical Noah, who in his ark played savior to all species of life at the physical level, saving them from the floods, the *avatar* is a savior to all life at the spiritual level. He saves them from the quagmire of materialism.

The *avatar* is the descent of Divinity into flesh. It is *aja* (unborn) so that it can never die. Normally, in spiritual evolution a *Paramahansanath Yogi* evolves to a *Siddhanath Yogi* who then further progresses to the evolutionary stature of an *Avadhootnath Yogi*. He is then the beacon of spiritual light to the world, unfettered and free. He is the "enlightened swan" flying high and soaring beyond the limited comprehension of mortal man. Being supremely free, he has no *karma* to fulfill and attains to the final *Niranjana Nirvana*. Having merged into the Supreme Divinity, he returns to the world no more. But if he does return under very rare circumstances, fully robed with the Light and Love of God, he comes for a world liberating mission. Then and only then may he be said to be the *Avatarnath Yogi*.

The classical and well-known *avatar*s are Rama, Krishna, and Buddha. The work of the *avatar* is to protect the righteous, to destroy all negativity and darkness, and to establish the *dharma* of right living. They come from age to age. Gyanavatar Shri Yukteswar, in his book, *"The Holy Science,"* has clearly given the length and duration of the four human *yugas* or ages, as being different from the four celestial ages. The first two ages are *Satya Yuga* (golden age of 4800 years), followed by the *Treta Yuga* (the silver age of 3600 years). Then comes the *Dwapara Yuga* (copper age of 2400 years.) Finally comes the dark age of *Kali Yuga* (Iron age of 1200 years). The coming of these lofty Beings of Truth, and the periods in which they incarnate, has also been mentioned in the *Baghavad Gita*. The *avatar* incarnates at the most needed hour of humanity.

In the case of Shiva-Goraksha-Babaji, he is a *Swayambhoo*, also called a *Mahavatar*. This shall be explained later.

The Divine Signs of a True Avatar

a. The body of an *avatar* is composed by *Kriya Shakti* of pure spiritual light and is not subject to disease, decay or death. This body of light is beyond the ravages of time. On occasion, the *avatar* casts no shadow.

b. The footprints of an *avatar* are not impressed on the seashore or the sands of causation and time, because he has no *karma* (deed), only *akarma* (divine work).

c. The birth of an *avatar* is not bound by *karma*, but he chooses it by divine will, whatever the manner of birth may be. Whether it is through the womb of a mother, by immaculate conception, or birth in a lotus, it is the divine will of the *avatar* free from *karma*. A divine *avatar* has the capacity to pull over himself the veil of cosmic illusion and incarnate into the world of mortal beings. It is a divine descent, being in the world of matter and *maya*, and yet not of it.

d. Resurrection. The *avatar*'s body is composed of divine, undecayable light. It has the capacity to die and then transform the atomic cells into a transfigured body of light, resurrecting itself to show the glory of the lord most high on the earth of mortal man. Resurrection is the special feature of the *avatar* alone. People who claim to be *avatars*, but who are incapable of resurrecting their bodies after death, are spiritually evolved beings of a lesser stature—they cannot be classified or called *avatars*. They may be saints, yogis, *Hamsas* and *Paramhamsas*.

The Different Types Of Avatars

The Mahavatar (Swyambhoo). This is specifically the great unborn, Self-manifestation of Shiva and has a much loftier work than the *avatar*. The Cosmic Being called Babaji-Gorakshanath will not incarnate from age to age, but is perpetually present until the world cycle is over. He broods over humanity, his children, from eternity to eternity. His work is far beyond the comprehension of mortals. He stands at the ninth level of Cosmic Consciousness.

Avatars of Shiva. Also called the manifestations of Lord Shiva, the *Shiva Kumars*. Standing at the eigth level of Cosmic Consciousness, they are usually invisible and unknown. However, they incarnate specifically for the yogic and spiritual evolution of human consciousness. They are not limited to the *yuga* cycle as are the *avatars* of Vishnu, but manifest when the need of spiritual evolution arises. They are also called the *Agnishvatta Rishis* (the Sages of the Fire Mist).

Avatars of Vishnu. These are the classic *Avatars* at the seventh level of Cosmic Consciousness who come for the salvation of mankind from age to age according to the yuga cycle. They are in order, Matsya (fish), Kaccha (tortoise), Varaha (boar), Narsimha (man-lion), Waman (dwarf), Parshu Rama (ancient man), Rama (perfect man), Krishna (divine man), Buddha (enlightened man) and Kalki (divine Savior). These incarnations not only signify the physical evolution, but evolve the consciousness of all humanity as well.* The last three are Purna Avatars.

Purna Avatars (complete descent of Divinity in human body). The *Purna Avatar* is that consciousness of Divinity, which descends in the haunts of human beings to establish righteousness and spiritually evolve human consciousness. This God-made-flesh comes to Earth every *yuga*. Krishna, the Buddha, and the Kalki are ideal examples of the *Purna Avatar*. The last is yet to incarnate in the world at the junction of the Leo-Aquarius age. These beings are at the eigth level of Cosmic Consciousness.

---

* In my observation, a similar evolutionary process of the ten *Avatars* is replayed at a lower human scale in the womb of a mother. Here the embryo first appears as the fish avatar, then the tortoise, the boar-faced, then man-lion, then the miniscule dwarf, then the human achetype (Parshuram), then the human form receiving sensations (Ram), then emotions (Krishna), then the developed embryo receiving ideations from the mother (Buddha). Finally the fetus is fully evolved, ready to be born into a whole new consciousness, which represents the Kalki Avatar.

***Aunsh Avatars*.** This is the partial *avatar* which manifests for the evolution of all human souls. The partial *avatar*, like the full *avatar*, has already attained to *Nirvana Moksha*, the seventh level of Cosmic Consciousness. The difference between the two is that the partial *avatar*, when descended on earth, manifests only a part of his Divinity commensurate with his work. The nature of his work on earth needs him to manifest only so much of his Divine Consciousness as can complete his mission. The full *avatar* has no such limitations.

I am bringing to light that the *Avatars of Vishnu* are considered to be his direct emanation through one of the seven primeval flames, called the Seven *Rishis* of the ancient of days, the archangels of the heavenly host and collectively the sacred Elohim of eternal living fire. Lord *Krishna*, for example, was a direct emanation of *Sanatana Rsi Naryana*. He is, however, the descent of Deity in form (*mayavi rupa*) of individuality. His appearance to man on earth is objective but in sober fact is not so. His illusive form has no past or future, nor does he have reincarnations due to *karma*, which has no hold on him.

The consciousness of all *avatars* is fully enlightened, far beyond the comprehension of humans, totally and wholly merged into the Absolute. Pulling the veil of the cosmic illusion, it creates for itself what is called a *mayavi roop*, meaning an illusionary idea body composed of the three *gunas* of *sattva* (luminosity), *rajas* (activity), and *tamas* (inertia). Then the Divine materializes the radiant astral body, which ultimately forms a physical body that can appear and disappear at will. The divine body of congealed light casts no shadow and no footprints. It is the divine light in a material world.

The work and mission of the *avatar* has been explained above and the details of the *Kalki,* our coming Messiah, will be given now.

The Kalki Avatar and His Assistants

The coming of the Kalki Avatar is also called the second advent, or by some, Judgment Day. This is the time when all people shall be judged according to their karma and perfect justice meted out. Negativity itself shall be punished, and goodwill and peace shall rule the earth. Mighty shall be the descent of these Beings in their chariots of spiritual fire. It is to be remembered that when so supernal and lofty a Being as Kalki, descends on earth he is a *Purna Avatar*, that is a full *Avatar* (for details refer to the *Bhavishya Purana* and *Kalki Purana*).

The *Kalki Avatar* will be accompanied by two mighty assistant *Avatar*s. The first will be the *Manu Savarni* whom people know as the King Vikramaditya (victorious Sun). Some know him as El Morya and to some he is known as the Divine Sisodia Gulablal Singh. But there is a mystery in this, which try as we may, we cannot resolve. Hence, we are not making the endeavor to do so. However, this is the ideal king who will be accompanying the lofty Kalki Avatar. Also accompanying him will be the divine Priest who was in his former lives the King Devapi mentioned in the classic Indian epic *Mahabharata*. Devapi was also known as the Rishi Koothumi who is destined to be the spiritual preceptor and World Teacher.

The Mahavatar Babaji and His Assistants

The doctrine of the Avatar unfolds as we study the ancient scriptures of India. The *Kalki Purana*, the *Bhavishya Purana* and the *Chandogya Upanishad* give us fascinating insights into the nature of this Divine Shiva Kumar, loftier in spiritual stature than even the *Purna Avatar*. "There He stood, 'The Youth of Sixteen Summers,' Sanata Kumar, the 'Eternal Virgin Youth,' the new ruler of the world, come to his kingdom, His pupils, the three *Rudra Kumars* with Him, His helpers around Him; thirty mighty Beings, great beyond Earth's reckoning, in graded order, clothed in the glorious bodies they had created by *Kriya Shakti*. This was the first spiritual hierarchy."

Some of the lofty *Rudras* (aspects of Shiva), of his hierarchy are Sanatana, Sanandana, Sanaka-Sujata, Lord Dakshinamurti, Lord Dattatreya, Adi-Shankaracharya, Buddha, Christ, Hermes, Patanjali, Lord Kalki Maitreya, Lord Vaivashvat Manu, Lord Parshuram, and Yogavatar Lahiri Mahasaya. In the next echelon we have the *Chiranjeevs* ("Immortals"), Karna/ El Morya Vikramaditya (the one who is to succeed the Divine King, Vaivashvat Manu), Devapi/Naga Arjuna (the one who is to succeed the World Teacher, Kalki Maitreya), Lord Hanuman, Ashvathama, Arjuna, Aaryasangh /Jwala Kula ("family flame"), Count St.Germain, Bali, and Gyanavatar Yukteshwar.

The celestial manifestation of Shiva-Goraksha-Babaji appeared on earth eighteen-and-a half-million years ago at the begining of the *Vaivashvat Manvantar*, the duration of the reign of the seventh spiritual king, Vaivashvat Manu. There are fourteen such *Manus* in one *kalpa* or *day of Brahma*. We are currently in the middle of the *Shveta Varaha Kalpa* (World Cycle of the White Boar). He is now the silent Watcher who directs all *Avatars* and Prophets in their evolutionary work and mission. The deeper nature of his own work is beyond our comprehension.

The *Linga Purana* was taken from India by Buddhist monks and is worshipped in great secrecy in the chief monasteries in Tibet and Nepal. Shiva-Goraksha-Babaji, this deathless Presence of eternity, keeps in his aura even the coming of the Kalki Avatar and all of the manifestations Divine. It is not given to us to know what arrangement for a spiritual impetus to humanity shall be given at the beginning of the new millennium, but it is said that a tremendous Being, a manifestation of Shiva Babaji himself shall incarnate at the end of the millennium in one or many souls and do as great a work on the spheres of the inner consciousness of humanity as the Kalki Avatar will do on the outer consciousness of humanity.

A galvanic spiritual impetus shall come from this manifestation of Shiva. This evolutionary surge given by this lofty Being called the *Mahavatar* is to avoid the dire consequences of wiping out humanity from the face of the earth while spiritually enabling it to take the paradigm shift so glibly talked about by parrots of the parlor. Of course, the great Babaji, The Presence, will ever be a silent witness to this divine drama.

Divine Workers and Assistants the World Over

In order to assist the massive surge of spiritual change, we the *Hamsa Yoga Sangh* must take our stand under the great *Siddha Sangha*, which is the Guardian Wall of Humanity. We must serve humanity as our larger Self and dedicate ourselves to the furthering of human awareness by teaching the *Babaji Kriya Yoga*. We must enable everyone to experience the unified field of consciousness, thus making all human beings realize that at the level of consciousness Humanity is One—so that we may all live on this planet in peaceful co-existence. This would enable people to take the quantum leap into the Great Reality when the ever-present Babaji Gorakshanath gives that Truth, and to later flow in the evolutionary process of love and joy when the Kalki Avatar comes at the beginning of the Leo-Aquarius Age.

The Avadhoot/Avatar Doctrine

The difference between an *avatar* and an *avadhoot* is that the *avatar* is the involution of the Divine into the human and the *avadhoot* is the evolution of the human into the Divine. The *avadhoot* literally means "cast-off." He has shaken off all worldly ties and concerns; the highest renunciate ever-absorbed in Supreme Consciousness. He is a yogi who has crossed the 6th degree of initiation, meaning that even the last vestiges of his *karma* of stored impressions have been worked out.

He, the Conscious Seer, in *nirbija samadhi*, is totally free from the seed of the mind and matter of the universe. The cycle of birth and death ceases for him and *karmic* desire cannot pull him down to reincarnate on earth unless he chooses to do so. However, when he does reincarnate, it is as a savior, a partial *avatar*.

One of the prevailing views about a soul who has evolved to the stature of an *avadhoot* through a series of incarnations and accumulated merit is that his meditations and good *karma* cannot make him a *Nirvani*, but can lead him to a Divine *Sat-Guru*. Then by the Guru's grace, he will be initiated into the mysteries of *Niranjana Nirvana* and attain to Divine union. The other view is that from our works alone we obtain *moksha*, and if we take no pains there will be no gains—grace from the Deity (*Maha Guru*) does not come to the lazy. In order to procure the grace of the Guru, the disciple must make the initial effort. Therefore it is maintained that the Buddha, though an *avatar* in one sense, is a true *Param-mukta Avadhoot*. Owing to his personal merit and endeavor, he attained *Nirvana* and is more cherished than an *avatar*.

My personal view is that both individual effort in Yoga and devotion bring about the grace of the Guru, which is necessary to achieve the blessed state of *Nirvana Moksha*. The grace of God and Guru, like the sun, shines equally on all beings because in the eyes of the Divine, all are equal, and the God-essence is no respecter of personal egos. Grace is planted as conscience in the minds of each of us and it is we who bring about the grace and disgrace of God in our lives, by either hiding in the dark room of karmic negativity or exposing ourselves to sunshine of divine grace through good deeds. We are responsible for the grace of God in our lives and disgrace of ourselves by our own deeds. Only past life effort of good works makes it appear as grace in this life because we have no memory recall of the past. The truth is that a particular Soul that appears to be graced by the Divine has already made the effort in a past or present life.

Incarnations and Rebirths

There is a very subtle difference between a partial *avatar* and an *avadhoot*. In fact, in terms of Self-Realization they have both attained *moksha*. The difference is that the *avadhoot* does not enter his entire causal and spiritual consciousness into *Nirvana Moksha*. He makes his spiritual self (*atma*) experience the wisdom of *nirvana* while keeping his causal body intact to reincarnate as a savior of humanity with this same causal body. From this later evolved the *Bodhisattva* doctrine of Indian Buddhism. On the other hand, the partial *avatar* merges his all into *Nirvana Moksha*. His causal body and *atma* are both transformed and resolved into *Brahma Nirvana* (*Nirvana Moksha*). To sum it up, we can say that an *avadhoot* who enters *Nirvana Moksha* never returns and if he does he comes as a partial *avatar*.

For the sixth degree initiates, the next question is this: if an *avadhoot* purifies his causal body to the extent of having no residual *karma* in it, then the causal body, as per the *Advaita Vedanta* philosophy, shall resolve in pure consciousness. Hence, in order to incarnate on the terrestrial plane, he involutes to pull around himself a vesture composed of sub-atomic particles of light, creating this veil of *maya* by his own yogic power (*kriya shakti.*) This is the *mayavi* or illusionary body of light that he can use to incarnate when needed.

The other option he has is to keep that slender film of causal body of good *karma* to enable him to reincarnate for the salvation of humanity. The fifth degree process of *Jivan Mukta* is that he is one level lower than the *avadhoot* and has not dissolved his pure body film.

Rebirths may be classified into three categories:

- Divine incarnations called *Avatarnaths*.
- Adepts who forego *Nirvana* to help humanity (*avadhootnaths*)
- Natural rebirths as per law of *karma* (ordinary people)

In very exceptional rebirths, the high initiate *Avadhoot*, before disappearing in *Nirvana Moksha*, can, for reasons best known to him, cause his body of causal light to remain behind. Not being an *avatar*, he is a knower (an Enlightened Being). The *Avadhoot* has achieved *Nirvana Moksha*, but chooses not to enter that final state, remaining instead on our planet for the salvation of humankind.

A lower degree of incarnation, that of a *Siddha (aulia)*, is able to transfer the memory of his past life to his body with traces of it to be worked out. These traces may be a result of having taken on the *karma* of some of his disciples.

In the third degree, a practicing *Hamsa Yogi*, who has passed on from this life to the next, would, commensurate with his *karma*, choose a suitable body and circumstances in that incarnation to progress in his spiritual evolution, but in most cases would lose all memory of his previous incarnation.

The most intriguing mystery of the *avadhoot* lies in the fact that how—when his consciousness is in *Nirvana*—does his causal body associate with the astral desire body of one of his worthy disciples? And how does he work out the latter's *karma* to give the disciple blessings in the form of an evolutionary boost?

Usually this initiate to whom such a blessing is given is called a *"mast"* (*musth*) meaning "divinely mad". They are God-intoxicated by an excessive surge of *Kundalini* energy, which they cannot handle nor use to further their evolution. Such a state is also called a state of *khumari*. This *avasta* (state) occurs during the process of *kundalini* awakening, anywhere between 3rd degree initiate of a *Hamsanath Yogi* and the 4th degree of *Paramahansanath Yogi* right up to the *Siddhannath Yogi*. This divinely intoxicated state of undirected spiritual energy is found more commonly among the *bhakti* devotees and *Sufi* mystics. It occurs because of a lack of the complete system of yogic techniques to safely channelize the *kundalini* energy to the state of a successful *nirvikalpa samadhi*.

The *Avadhoot* and *Avatar* Personalities

Gajanan Maharaja from the village of Shaegaon (India) was a 19th century *avadhoot* who helped a lesser *mast* initiate to such a degree that he himself appeared to be the *mast*, but in fact was assisting his disciple to work out his karma by actually wearing the astral body of the disciple. Besides this he had also worked with many normally evolving students as well. The enlightened *avadhoot* takes it upon himself to empower his student from a *mast*-intoxicated state of a *savikalpa samadhi* to a *nirvikalpa samadhi*. Holding back one's own entry into *Brahma Nirvana* for the sake of younger souls to come—surely, a divine way of serving humanity as one's larger Self.

Sainath of Shirdi in Maharastra (India) is one of the greatest enigmas in the spiritual hierarchy of *Nath Yogis*. He behaved exactly like an *avadhoot* but in the reality showed all the signs of an *avatar*. His raising the dead, casting no shadow from his body on occasions, and himself appearing in resurrected rainbow body of light, leads me to realize the *avataric* stature of this *Nath Yogi*. At the same time, his losing body consciousness and falling down, behaving like a *mast* and losing control of his body, makes one think he is an *avadhoot* deeply involved in assisting many divinely intoxicated yogis and *Sufis* to evolve along the spiritual path. Since this great being also helped in the spiritual evolution and *karmic* dissolution of normal initiates and people, *Sainath* is truly the most mystic of the modern-era of *avatars*. The *avatar* takes on the furthering of human awareness in deeper dimensions of Consciousness.

Gyannath (*Jnaneswar*) "The Avatar of Wisdom" was born in the village of Alandi (Maharashtra, India) in the 13th century. He is called the king of mystics by the high initiates of the secret circles of the

Nath Mandala. His *Maha Guru* was Babaji-Gorakshanath himself, who initiated the young Gyannath into the mysteries of *Nath Yoga* and the ultimate realization of *nirvikalpa* and *sanjeevan samadhi*. Having successfully accomplished the *Nath* yogic practices, he however found them too demanding for the normal people and householders. As a result he advocated the simple devotional pathway to God. From this evolved the *bhakti* tradition of the *Varkaris*. His miracles were not intended to aggrandize his spiritual stature, but to instill faith in the Divine into the hearts and minds of the then skeptical masses. However, his *mahasamadhi* also known as the *sanjeevan samadhi* (*saroub samadhi*), meaning the preservation of his rainbow-body of light in life and death, clearly points to his *Nath* knowledge. This more than shows us his *avataric* stature and mission, that not only is his Consciousness immortal, but the body and mind too—a distinct feature of immortality of the *Siddha-Nath* yogic tradition.

Mahavatar Babaji, "the Lord of Irradiant Splendor," is also called *Sanata Kumar*, meaning "the eternal virgin youth". He came to be by direct manifestation from *Nilalohita Shiva* (blue void of absolute Consciousness) infused in Brahma who is *viraj-vach* (light-sound). Holding in his hands the evolutionary lightning of life and death, Babaji is called "*Vaidhatra*" meaning "the Cosmic Lightning Holder of Divine Destiny". This word (*vaidhatra*) also means, "first from the Creator". Accompanying Shiva-Goraksha-Babaji are thirty-three lofty beings, the *Shiva-Kumars*, the immortal virgin youths. Babaji is *Jagannath* (Lord of the Universe), the head of the spiritual hierarchy of the Sages of the Fire Mist with their rainbow bodies of light, all in graded order, to assist him in his divine evolutionary work. The *kumars* are the true progenitors of spirit in humanity and because of these incomprehensible beings, the holders of the sacred flame, the spiritual evolution of humanity was and is continuously made possible. In ancient texts, they incensed the *devas* (the celestial beings) for imparting the secrets of the Divine to mortal men. Wonderful accounts about this wondrous Being and his Divine assistants are given in the *Markandeya Purana*, and the *Samkhya Karika* of Ishvar Krishna.

Meeting With An Avadhoot

Talking of *avadhoots*, I have an interesting story to relate. I was, during my younger days, very fond of an Indian sweet called *jalebi*, and visited a simple roadside sweet shop (*dhaba*), where we dipped the freshly made hot *jalebis* in milk and ate them. A smiling mendicant used to visit the shop and his nonchalant appearance intrigued me. This carefree wanderer, with his eyes gazing out into the unknown, pretended to relish with us the sweets. He, however, was not aware of what he ate. Nor did he appear to possess his body, which hung loosely about his person. Many a person came to the sweet shop and the young ladies who visited the place would be teased by this stranger. Many passed him off as a mad man.

Then one day I saw him lying on the footpath near the shop. He had apparently been beaten up by some ladies and their men for teasing. I went close to him and a strange sight met my eyes. He was lying on the floor smiling, his head bleeding, and a far away voice from within his body asked, "Are you happy, have you had enough now or do you want some more?" I opened my eyes wider and immediately felt attracted to this being, so that night I searched out his hut. When I peeped into the hut, I was agog to behold a blue halo of light surrounding this being who, during the day, played out his drama of teasing girls. His body was breathless and as rigid as a rock lost in the splendor of *samadhi*. With the wings of light, he had fled to his Divine abode of Cosmic Consciousness (*Paramartha Satya*). His higher, real Self was in *Nirvana*, while the apparent body he had acquired was to assist some of his pupils in working out their *karma*. To show such love for a pupil is very mysterious, an aspect of the Master - pupil relationship only understood between the two. He alone can explain why an *avadhoot* would do as he would do. So I closed my eyes and slid into my *dhyana* meditation—truly Oh Lord! Thy ways are and ever shall be incomprehensible to man.

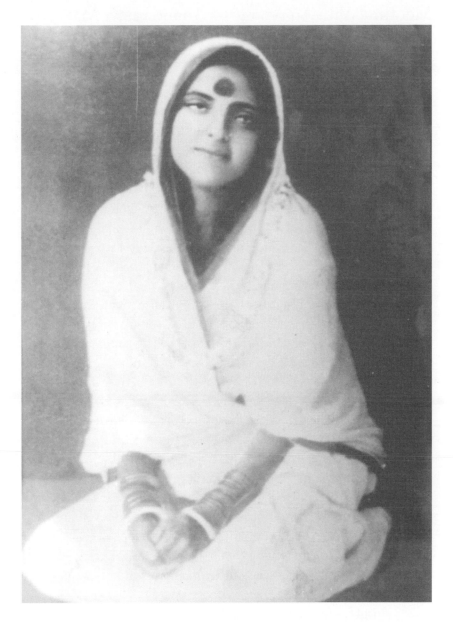

Anandamayi Ma: Prem Avatar of
the Divine Mother in Bhava Samadhi

Meeting With An Avatar — Anandamayi Ma

She was the bliss-permeated Mother. I had the good fortune to meet her on many occasions, and had many sweet memories in the aura of this Divine Being. One rainy afternoon I left home in haste. I was homesick and I wanted to be absorbed in her presence. On reaching her *ashram* in *Pune*, I found the door to her room closed. I did not want to disturb her but stood in the rain, my eyes transfixed on the door as if I would stare it open. It did open, but only after I had practiced rain yoga for twenty minutes or so, a mild *tapa* to wash away some negative *karma* before meeting with the Divine, I thought to myself.

She smiled and called me indoors saying I was a stubborn child, and so I was. Before I sat, I proceeded to touch her feet (which she normally does not permit), but as I touched her feet, I was shocked to find my hands go through her bones and flesh to touch the floor. My body was electrified at that. I remembered that an *Avatar* is an illusion of light in the illusion of the world. It can at will, to increase a person's faith, make one experience his or her body of light. No flesh, no shadow, no *karma*. How can a nobody have any *karma*? An *Avatar*ic Being is *karmaless*, when it does work in *maya*, it leaves no *samskaras*. It's like writing on water. When the unliberated student does his daily chores or work, he creates *karma*—it's like writing on the sand. Uplifted and wonder-struck by this experience, I settled in a trance-like state and saw her radiance flooding the whole *ashram* and countryside. As my body elongated, my Consciousness left it to expand and merge in her wondrous aura. I was blessed, and when I opened my eyes, the surroundings were still radiant with her presence. An hour later she said, "You are your own *Guru*, go and spread the word of the Lord in far lands," and went into *samadhi* again.

In all my travels and spiritual experiences, in all my meditations and direct experiences, the realization that has dawned on me is that *Anandamayi Ma* is the only woman *Avatar* of the century. She is often loosely and wrongly equated with popular modern women saints, *yoga* teachers, or others of similar names. We are blessed to have such Divine *Avatars* with us, without whom pure spirituality would have vanished from the face of this Earth long ago.

A Unique Feature of the Non-Dual Phenomena

We now go on to the most marvelous evolutionary happening in spiritual history: a non-dual *advaita* process—the most incomprehensible and awesome miracle between spirit and matter.

When the *kama sharir* or astral desire body of a high initiate is left behind, it purifies itself by contact with its Divine *Rishi*, one of the nine flames of the Cosmic *Naths*. This sage helps the astral body to assimilate more of the intuitional nature and purity of mind. The astral desire body is then too pure to be dissolved in the astral plane, its intermediate state between two incarnations. It lives on to evolve towards purity and finds its own degree of salvation in a wisdom body, which then is assimilated in that celestial body. It then becomes itself the luminous star of the soul. This star introverts upon itself, turning itself inside out, to involute through its own Divine mind star-gate to vanishing point, and evolute to become infinite divine consciousness. How does it do that? The answer is by the *Rishi Guru's* grace, which is reciprocating the mind-star's right endeavor. In scientific parlance, the *gurutva akarshan* (intense gravitational attraction) of the *Rishi Guru* pushes the mind-star* out of four-dimensional existence into a Self-Realized Consciousness.

---

*Lord *Maitreya* will inhabit the causal mind-star of Purna Avatar Krishna to re-incarnate as the Kalki Avatar and complete his mission as the next savior of all sentient and non-sentient beings. The causal mind-star shall thereafter gravitate through its own star-gate and finally merge into infinite Consciousness. Presently, the Kalki-Maitreya is established in the Supreme Conscious ecstasy of Yoga with his Cosmic *Nath Guru*, the Brahma-Rishi Parashara, abiding in the bosom of duration until the commencement of the Leo-Aquarius age when he shall descend in flame and fire to establish righteousness amongst the people of the earth.

This is the story of the evolution of the astral desire body into the Soul Consciousness. A very rare happening because it defies both the *Samkhya* philosophy and the economy of nature.

Normally all bodies, physical, astral and causal, composed of the sub-atomic particles of *tama*, *raja* and *sattva gunas* resolve back into the transcendental matrix of the matter and mind of the universe. They do not transform to Divine Consciousness, as is the rare case of this non-dual *advaita* phenomena given above. This is one of the inexplicable mysteries of the *Avadhoot-Avatar* doctrine. So, what I'm saying is that in the case of the *Avadhoot* or *Avatar*, such a quantum leap of evolution is possible even for their cast-off astral bodies, once they associate with their Divine Being—the Cosmic *Naths*.

CHAPTER 15

SANATANA DHARMA
Earth Peace Through Self Peace

If earth peace is to herald the dawn of the new age, we must all realize that, **"Humanity is our uniting religion, Breath our uniting prayer, and Consciousness our uniting God."** Today, as responsible citizens of the world, we must find a lasting solution to dissolve our animosity and to bring about a peaceful co-existence among people and nations of the world.

So here we are with this beautiful formula, a philosophy for earth peace to be worked out by each of us individually and all of us collectively. Many believe it would bring about a commonality to the human family. But we are not sufficiently motivated to bring about the peace process through such a means. For this to happen, practical and dynamic pathways to peace must be formulated. Fortunately such simple pathways to peace and yogic meditations are already being taught at schools, public forums and meditative gatherings of *Hamsa Yoga Sangh*.

The teachings for peace are non-denominational and attract people from all over the globe, irrespective of their religion, caste or creed. Very dynamic and simple Earth Peace meditations are being taught to children and adults alike all over the world. I have also chartered a "Declaration of Human Rights for Earth Peace," which enables citizens of the world community to know and to practice the Earth Peace meditations, one of the important pathways to peace.

Humanity our uniting religion: This fact of truth is imperative to the understanding of all humanity if peaceful co-existence is to be realized. More for better than for worse our humanity of six billion two hundred million people is living on this planet. The basic question with which we must deal is:

How best may we utilize this vast human resource called Humanity for our own welfare, and for the evolution of our consciousness? What are the means we possess? What is the "connectus canarsus" of all human beings on this planet whereby we may unite to know our oneness?

That all human beings are "religioned" (bonded) by the commonality of being human is an undeniable fact. Hence humanity is one's uniting religion.

Breath our uniting Prayer is the next fact we must understand. Unless we can realize a common dynamic process we all participate in, we will not live peacefully. Breath is the common denominator of humanity and all living beings. It forms the "feel alike" brotherhood of humanity partaking of the same breath of life. If we can somehow make the human race aware of this sharing of a common breath, we can bring a great deal of harmony to the different faiths and religions of the world.

Therefore in order to make all people experience the sharing of the same breath, it becomes necessary to demonstrate it. This brings us to the first pathway to peace called *pranapat*. Here the *Master* Yogi, by his love, expands his *pranic* breath and infuses it into the breath of hundreds or thousands of truth seekers. Thereby their breath becomes longer, richer and deeper. This gives all who experience it an awareness of the unity of humanity. It also makes them aware that people are united by the sacred prayer of breath. Otherwise, nobody could breathe through their breath. This demonstrates that humanity is linked by the Self-same cord of breath.

The experience of *pranapat* is given to bring about a peaceful coexistence among people. This experience is also given to let humanity know that, "Breath is one's only prayer." If one does not pray to God for a few days he still survives, but if one does not live God (that is, if he does not breathe God), he dies. So vital is the breath aspect of God for our existence.

Consciousness our uniting God: Our existence is rooted in our consciousness. Untainted by any religion or ideologies, we come to the third and most vital understanding of our livingness factor. This is untainted by any man-made notions of God, and free from the pride and prejudices of each religion claiming to be the truest. Here we come to the third and most vital understanding of our livingness; the still silence within us, called consciousness, is the parent source of all humanity. Its Supra-consciousness glory is the *raison-d'etre* of all human existence and evolution. Consciousness is the inner drive and motivating factor not only of human evolution but its genius and material progress too. Without the spark of enthusiasm from this inner consciousness, humanity would have remained a senseless shell. To awaken to our reality is to awaken to our Consciousness, our uniting God!

With this understanding in view, I felt the burning need to express my consciousness to the people at large. I came up against the barrier of the mind. This was my first obstacle—I could express my mind by writing books and by giving talks, but the question was, how can I express my no-mind consciousness? Certainly it was not through words or letters. Then came my profound experience with Babaji, by whose grace I was able to give all receptive seekers an experience of my Soul Consciousness of thoughtless awareness. This experience led me to my work on the "Unified Field of Consciousness"—that, if one Consciousness is bereft of thought in soulful awareness, then all other minds attuned to that Consciousness shall be identically transformed to it. This affirms my vision for earth peace: "At the level of Consciousness, Humanity is One." I call the giving of this experience *Shivapat*.

Laying out a clear and succinct direction for our *Hamsa* students was important. Hence, the mission statement for our non-profit organization, the *Hamsa Yoga Sangh*, became:

We, the *Hamsas*, servants of Humanity, are
Meditated to the furthering of Human Awareness
Dedicated to serving Humanity as our Larger Self
Devoted to new life awakenings for Earth-Peace healing through Self-Peace healing.

Students learn and meditate with the *acharyas* (teachers) of this movement. Then they set out as servants of humanity for their own work. The mission statement is clear in their minds. They then endeavor to actualize their mission for Earth-peace through Self-peace.

Meditating to further human awareness, they apply themselves to the expansion of that peaceful consciousness to ever more widening groups of both peace-loving and aggressive people. They also endeavor to spread the consciousness of peaceful co-existence to all faiths, and to all organizations that disrupt peace. The vibrations of the strong "Intent of Peace" are exploded into the minds of terrorists and aggressive people too. This is most effective during the full moon "Earth Peace meditations". Thereby the obstacles toward the evolution of human consciousness are removed. Consequently the meditation to further human awareness goes on.

Dedicated to serving humanity as our larger Self, the person must put service before self. He must sacrifice his smaller pleasures to first serve the larger Self. Upon doing so, the spiritual aspirant begins to experience an indescribable joy flowering within himself. He is so engrossed in the sorrows of others that he forgets his own little sorrows. He becomes a storehouse of bliss, radiating to others.

The servant of humanity is so absorbed in seeing to the needs of others that he forgets his own. He then is not in any need. He neither craves nor wants anything, becoming a fully satisfied storehouse of giving. Oh what a joy to serve the Lord disguised as the suffering humanity. How honored is a servant of humanity to be able to do this. And finally one's own evolution is quickened and enhanced by the selfless work.

Devoted to new life awakening for Earth Peace healing through Self-Peace healing, the *Hamsa* servant applies himself to the third mission statement. This may be done in a thousand and one ways. The most effective way is to impart to an ailing society the healing joy of God, by teaching Earth Peace meditations. Food, medicine and clothing are also essential factors in bringing about equanimity and peace in third world nations. Large multi billion dollar foundations must be made aware of the virtue of giving if goodwill and peace are to prevail on earth more effectively.

The Declaration Of Human Rights For Earth Peace is to make us citizens of the world more aware of ourselves. Detailed next is what is ours by birthright.

During the course of my *sadhana* (spiritual practice), I was inspired by Babaji to develop techniques to boost the inward journey of the Soul. To further the noble cause of *Sanatana Dharma*, I give the *Shivapat* and *Pranapat*.

DECLARATION OF HUMAN RIGHTS FOR EARTH PEACE

If Earth Peace is to herald the Dawn of the New Age, realize "The Soul Cry" :
Humanity Our Uniting Religion
Breath Our Uniting Prayer and
Consciousness Our Uniting God!

To serve Humanity as our Larger Self by Earth Peace meditation on full moon days, absorbing its peaceful rays within while radiating them to the world without.

Use the way of the Peaceful Breath, which flows equally in all, as a means for attaining Earth Peace, thereby diffusing individual and international conflicts.

One's inalienable right lies in the furthering of the **Evolution of Human Consciousness** for World Peace, by exercising your will to good for making one another's lives on this planet a celebration.

By virtue of being a World Citizen, it is One's inborn right to attain the **Consciousness of Natural Enlightenment** leading to the realization that your expanded consciousness and humanity's consciousness is One.

As we evolve, we live less and less in our bodies and more and more in our consciousness. Hence, fusion of your positive awareness with that of nature's cultivates an improved and balanced eco-system. **Help to evolve Nature with your Nature, because Nature is the Nature of Man!**

Allow yourself to heal and be healed of the negativity of your mind by letting go of the negative mind, which covers the splendor of your Soul.

Shivapat: Unified Field of Consciousness

Shivapat - the *Satguru* gives his Soul Consciousness of thoughtless awareness experience to the disciple. I will now discuss with you the way he gives his Soul. This is the true essence of what he gives to demonstrate his love. So when you go anytime to see a true Master or *Satguru*, these are the qualities that you should see. If they cannot give you of themselves, then they fall short in their love for humanity; they are not a *Satguru*. They may be your beloved, your brother or maybe a Guru, but they are not the *Satguru*. The true Master gives you his Soul awareness.

Definition of my Philosophy: *The Satguru does not transmit Shivapat, but he, as Consciousness, awares himself into the mind-disciple, transforming that mind into his own Consciousness to the degree of the disciple's receptivity to the Master. In turn, the disciple's mind, attuned to the undifferentiated Consciousness of his Master, shall gravitate itself out of light-mind existence, to aware itself into that Consciousness, to the degree of its attunement with that Consciousness.*

Shivapat is another word for, "the sharing of *samadhi*," but only in a certain sense. How much you take of the experience of his Soul depends upon your spiritual evolution. Does he do this for recompense or to prove that he is something? No. He does it in all humility, as a servant of humanity. When I do it, I mentally bow to you as a sleeping image of God or partially awakened essences of God, and then I give you my Knowingness. Another word for the Soul is Divine Consciousness, or still awareness.

So the true Master should not only be in a state of Divine Consciousness and still awareness, but he must also be able to transfer and give unto receptive disciples this Divine Consciousness, this experience of his still Soul. All of you who have been with me, have privately and publicly experienced this "contentless" consciousness of thoughtless awareness by the grace of the Divine.

You know that all human beings want the best. They don't want the second best thing, even in this spiritual endeavor. That is their quality. But how much they persevere depends on them; it is a quality to be tested here. That they like the best is a good quality, which they aspire to, and why not? But then accompanied with that should be perseverance.

When the stillness is given by the Master to the disciple, there are three grades and stages of receptivity that the disciple may have. First, those whose conscious, subconscious, and super-conscious minds are totally open and in tune with the Master's, they get a complete stillness. They experience his Soul, but just the still Consciousness part of it. They do not experience anything in their senses like a sweet taste, the smell of jasmine, or a rose. They do not experience ecstasy in the first stage. They must meditate ceaselessly for God-bliss and cultivate it for themselves.

Then there are extended spiritual states, in which they do not hear anything. It's just a profound stillness of the Master's Soul, which is given to the disciple in that moment of time whereby he knows, along with the Master, the facticity of things. The facticity, rather, of Truth as it is. And that is not concerned with materialism. It's not the table nor the chair nor the television nor the bench nor our bodies. At that time, we may be aware of everything, but we do not associate with anything.

We can hear the child shouting in the road; we can see the television; we can hear the music but ah, Stillness is with us. We are not involved in the outer noise, so it doesn't associate with that. The Truth is immaterial. It is the direct experience of the Spirit of God, the Holy Spirit. I'm sure you appreciate and understand what I'm talking about, because I'm not talking about it, I'm just translating your experience into words. You have already experienced the Stillness of Soul Awareness.

A second group are those who are less receptive and have a little more closed mind (when I say mind, I refer to subconscious, conscious and super-conscious minds). These dear ones who are less receptive, will nevertheless experience a still center, which their thoughts cannot penetrate. We usually deal with the super-conscious mind here which enables the Soul to enter the bodies of other people, the Soul of the *Satguru*, his Divine Consciousness. We are not speaking of psychology here, nor are we speaking of parapsychology. We are not speaking of metaphysics or transpersonal psychology. We are speaking of this—the silence, the peace that passeth all understanding, which has no words, which is beyond all psychologies, which is Divine Consciousness. That is the union of the finite with the infinite Awareness.

A third group of people, whose minds are closed by stress or medication, experience the slowing down of their thoughts. They experience an awareness of thoughts moving slowly through their centers.

This is what the Master gives to the disciple in that moment of time, arresting the aging process of his body cells in that moment of time, preventing disease, decay and death. This is the Love that the *Satguru* has for his disciples. These are guidelines of how you may proceed along the spiritual path and know who is what. And then ultimately the *Divya Guru*s or the *Avatars* come, who just give a touch or by their presence send you into *samadhi*. These are guidelines to help you walk the spiritual path of Truth. A sincere student avails of three virtues when experiencing *Shivapat*, the Soul consciousness. They are firstly, that it retards the aging process. Secondly, it validates to each individual that at the level of consciousness, humanity is one, and finally gives one the realization of his Divine indweller.

The law of macrocosm and microcosm (*Pinda Brahmanda*) states that, "as in the universe so in the human beings." In his astral *chakras* are located planetary *karma*. By working on them he may disengage himself from *karma* and the trammels of worldly involvement.

Therefore, to know the infinite Creator, the infinite Lord, we *yogically* teach you to, "Stop your minds. Stop! Peace be still." And there was a great calm. And Shiva Goraksha gave unto each of his disciples the capacity to still the storm of their minds' thoughts and evolve their consciousness. Not only did he give us the capacity to still our minds, but he gave the *Satguru* the capacity to still and evolve the minds of his disciples also. I am talking about something you all have experienced here. What I say is not alien to you, but it is home to you because you have experienced and had a taste of it. My thought is that if one mind becomes tranquil consciousness, all minds that are receptive will also become a crystal pool of thoughtless awareness of soul knowing. At the level of Consciousness humanity is one.

Shaktipat

The *Satguru* also works with the triple Divine quality of light, vibration and sound in the heart center, transforming emotions to love. And those emotions that can be transformed, are transformed, while those that are too heavy to be transformed, and that are irreparable, are sucked in by the Guru, who works like his humbler physical counterpart of the circulatory system. In the spiritual circulatory system, through the positive arteries, he pumps in God's life blood and gives you the Truth of livingness and light. And from your psychic veins, he takes out your negativity, which cannot be transformed through your psychic veins, by drinking the poisons of the negativity of the disciples and later transforming them in himself. He works on them and then he puts that energy into the cosmic reservoir, which later can be apportioned to people in need—those who have poverty of energy, lack of self-esteem, guilt, fear and the likes.

Then the *Satguru*, working from the heart center and transforming all emotions to love, takes the love to the third eye center. He works in the third eye center giving the triple Divine quality (light, vibration and sound), the experience of the Holy Ghost. In this light, vibration, and sound that the *Satguru* or the true Master gives with his awakened *kundalini*, there are three qualities that happen—the Father, the Son and the Holy Ghost; which is which?

Which is the grossest out of the triple divine quality? That is the vibration. You know sometimes you feel a pulsation, a vibration and heat. That heat and vibration is the Chrestos, the holy Spirit.

Next you come to the Son, the Christ, which is the light sound. The vibration and heat of the Holy Spirit, the Chrestos, connects to the light and sound of the Christ. The sound that you hear in your right ear, is that which the Master causes you to hear by opening up your higher dimension, your heightened state of awareness. This is how he is helping the disciple to evolve, to develop extrasensory perceptions and to evolve into a higher consciousness.

And then comes the Christos. So you have the Chrestos, the Christ, and the Christos. The Chrestos is in the navel of every human being who is evolving. And the Christ is in the heart center—the King of Love, "my shepherd is whose goodness failest never." You know the lacking is from our side, not his. Even when the Master represents the good Lord, when he gives you a transmission, some feel it while some don't. Does it mean that he has held it from one and not the other? No. They are not receptive. So you have the Chrestos at the navel, Christ at the heart center and the Christos in the third eye center, which is the Divine light. Beyond the Christos is also the Nameless One, "He About Whom Naught May Be Said". And that is "The Lightless Light, which lights that Light, which lights the Light of All Our Souls". Now this is the way by which his *kundalini shaktipat* (the Divine transmission of the Holy Spirit) works on his disciples to help them to an expanded state of awareness, helping their spiritual evolution.

Pranapat

The third way in which the *Satguru* or rabbi (such as Jesus) helps his *shishyas* (disciples), is by helping them to breathe. He breathes through their breath. They've had ample experience of this. Because there is no way I can explain to you how I do it, and neither can you explain to me how I get inside there. But you, you, and you and all of you have experienced this. There are no words by which we can formulate any *modus operandi*—there are no callous or mechanical words to show how this is done. You could say it's done by love or by the intent of the Master to sincerely help his disciples because he wants them to taste of the nectar, which is beyond words, beyond description. And in his endeavor to share with his brethren, he does this sacrifice.

This is a great evolutionary work by yogis that has always gone unrecognized. Not that we want everybody to sing about it or recognize it, but people just don't understand the import of what is being given them, because it's years ahead of its time. No gadget has the power to do that, not your television, your mobile phone, or any computer hardware or software could just breathe through everybody. Only an exemplary human being who has tread the path with sincerity and would share the truth with his brothers can demonstrate this fact. And he would be in tune with you and connect with your breathing to relieve your stress and heal your negative *karma*.

The *prana* is intelligent life-force energy. It is the livingness of the breath as the mind in motion. It is liquid mind, aerial mind, that is, pneumatic mind. The *prana* has a "pneumonosity," has flow of breath. And when the life-breath flows in the spinal cord it tends to soothe your whole system at the physical level. It washes away stress and tension because, even logically, the central nervous system is what we are working with. When we move *prana* in the central nervous system, it invariably diffuses all your tension. It is because the afferent and efferent nerves that are connected with the central nervous system and the autonomous nervous system are connected to the spinal cord.

So when you breathe in the spinal cord and work it, the *prana* diffuses and relaxes your tension. This benefit is the least of them, because we are not the physical body. The physical body is merely a shadow of the Soul. The mind is the shadow of the Soul and the shadow of the mind is the body. So the body's just a facility, like you've worn your scarf or your dress—you just take it and throw it away. At death you just cast away the body and you take another body. I always encourage students to forget the fear of death and strive wholeheartedly to realize their Divinity within. ***Birth and Death are a Chapter in your Life Story. But You as the Immortal River of Livingness, Flow On!***

India's Gift to the Humanity

"INDIA WAS CHINA'S TEACHER IN RELIGION AND IMAGINATIVE LITERATURE AND THE WORLD'S TEACHER IN PHILOSOPHY... A TRICKLE OF INDIAN RELGIOUS SPIRIT OVERFLOWED TO CHINA AND INUNDATED THE WHOLE OF EASTERN ASIA."
Lin Yutang, author 'Wisdom of India'.

Not through trumpets nor clarion calls, but as silent as the morning dew, has India's gift of spiritual knowledge seeped into the hearts of humanity. The very people who conquered them by means of war themselves became the conquered by India's spirit of peace and philosophy of love. The mindset and courage of our people to sustain wave after wave of foreign invasion, and yet engulf them in our culture is unique amongst the peoples of the earth. As though this was not enough, India went on to teach humanity the ultimate lesson of peace. They broke the shackles of British rule and went on the win their political independence in 1947. This was done by the totally peaceful means called *satyagraha* - a non-violent reaction against injustice, returning love for hate. This unique political movement was headed by the Indian mahatma and saint, Mohandas Karamchand Ghandhi.

In its expertise in the evolution of spiritual consciousness, India stands second to none. Its deep yogic insights and profound philosophies have greatly influenced European, Asian and now, even Western thought. India dominated Tibet and China's[1] philosophy and culture for twenty centuries. The contemporary techniquesof today, such as pranic healing sudarshan kriya, tai-chi, chi-gung, and reiki are like little whirlpools and eddies in the great river of ancient Indian Yoga and Spirituality.

As early as 500BCE Bhognath was initiated into the Kundalini Kriya Yoga by the immortal Kal-agni Nath of Kashi, a holy city of Northern India. He belonged to the Nav-Nath tradition of yogis. He then took Nath yogic and healing knowledge to China where he was called Bo-yang and later as the legendary Lao-Tzu, he established the taoist movement in China and gave as a gift to the people the sacred Kundalini Yoga which went by the name of Yin-Yang Yoga. Yin stands for Shakti, the female divine principle, whle Yang is Shiva, the male divine principle. He taught them the balance of pranayama, that is Tai-Chi, by breathing to unite the two male-female principles atop the head and enter the golden yoga state of samadhi. Bhognath also taught thousands of Chinese disciples Tantra, the yoga of transformation of sexual to spiritual energy.

Later in 300CE, another Indian yogi, the Buddhist Patriarch Bodhidharma established the Shaolin temple in China. He established the Dhyana (Zen) school of Chinese and Japanese Buddhism. He also taught the martial art of Mushti Prahara, the technique to strike at the vital centers (marmasthana) and temporarily cripple the enemy, but specifically warned his diciples never to use these arts for aggressive purposes, only for self-defense. This later became the Shaolin Kung Fu, the Tai Chi Chuan and the Japanese Karate.

India has been the source of the sacred wisdom and healing knowledge to the whole world since time immemorial. This selfless service from the enlightened yogis has largely been erased, forgotten

290

or ignored by those peoples who have benefited so much spiritually, physically and culturally. However, during historical times, there have survived records of the spiritualizing impact of these selfless yogis.

In the present time, there is an East-West exchange, for the West values nothing that is free, and so the compassionate Shiva-Goraksha-Babaji has decreed that there should be an exchange of Western material wealth for India's spiritual wealth. In all my travels the world over, I have realized that in spite of its shortcoming, India is the spiritual dynamo of the world. It shall lead humanity in wisdom's ways more and more as time flows on.

One of the wonderful gifts that India has given to the world is its yogic philosophy of death. The body is the apparent perishable self and the soul is the immortal self . When a body gets old, it is cast off like a worn out garment. The Soul lives on to transmigrate into a new-born body and family which will help it to work out its remaining karma. This philosophy of putting in its proper place one's mistaken identity has greatly eliminated the fear in the hearts of countless generations of peoples all over the world. It has given them a purpose to live for and a purpose to die, with courage and confidence, knowing that:

They're not this house of flesh and bones
Which sleeps decays and dies
They are immortal Consciousness
Lord of the Earth and Skies

Here is a poem on death as a stargate to the Divine:

Stargate Death

Why do people think of me
What I am not supposed to be
Death's cold hand they often say
Will snatch away your earthly stay

They call me Death and yet
I take them to Eternity
Oh this paradox of ignorance
Deludes humanity

Men steeped in earthly ignorance
Do dread me as their foe
Knowing not that to their Souls
The Star of Truth I show

Then shun me not ye mortal men
But Maya's dream decline
She binds you to mortality
I to Eternal Life sublime

Rejoice then when I come to you
Each time at end of life
It is to take you in my arms
From worldly storms and strife

Then with great lovingness and care
I'll put you at His feet
Beseech of Him your psychic ego
Never to repeat

Such are my humble services
I offer to mankind
Do I do this for recompense?
No, it's just my Love that's blind

This would be a great help to people in overcoming their fear of death. I am giving here the true picture of what death is. This is true education, not information, because I wrote this with a thoughtless mind. I had no mind. I was just aware. I was inspired and I flowed. And the pen glowed and the writing was carrying on. What a wonderful life; what sacrifice and love for all.

However, there are people called *Rishis* and *yogis* in the Himalayas who are giving love of a much higher quality by nature of which we breathe. They are breathing our breath for us. I have demonstrated and shown to those who attend my *satsangs* worldwide that Masters can breathe through your breathing. So how much more could the Grand Masters do? How much more would the Divine Masters do? It gives you reason to think sincerely and intently and inwardly from your Soul (not from your mind), but to knowingly know that this is the Truth, because you have experienced a Master breathing through your breath. Am I right? So that is the form of love that is given. This does not mean that those unknown Great Masters, away from the sight of mortal human beings are not great in their greatness. Their song was never sung on this earth and yet they are dying for us. By their every breath they give us New Life Awakening.

My experience during the course of my meditations and work is that the awareness of one's being can be applied in day-to-day work. The mind is unnecessary. It must be trained to lie subservient to the higher consciousness in all of us, and used only when called upon by the *yogi* or individual person, for thinking or planning one's way of life. A vigilant consciousness, free from interfering thoughts, can be used to read or write and do one's day-to-day work. All my poems in *Anubhuti* were written in a still-mind all-awareness state.

The difference between *unmani* (vigilant awareness) and *sahaj samadhi* (natural state of enlightenment) is of degree and not of kind. The *sahaj samadhi* is a more advanced state. The *avasta* or state of vigilant awareness or passive alertness, free of all thoughts, produced the best results in my work. This is because the mind is so clear it transforms to become pure awareness. The mind shall soon become obsolete and the future means of absorbing knowledge, I feel, will be through the *unmani* (no mind) awareness. Awareness is in the present and a direct means of experiencing knowledge. We must change the Gestalt and become the awareness, and as soon as this is done, the mind, with its train of thoughts, is dissolved. The thinking mind is an obstacle to the inflow of higher gnosis and Truth because its analytical and judgmental thought ripples distort the true message of the incoming knowledge. Only a consciousness, free from the ripples of thought in the mind's lake, can experience Divinity in all its splendor, all its beauty and all its Truth.

Because people are reluctant to leave their old habits that have made a home in the mind, I know they shall vehemently oppose this Truth, but we must take the quantum leap into the brave new world.

How can western authors with a minds colored by thought, judge a colorless mind, a contentless consciousness of a pure vigilant awareness? It can't be done because judgmental thoughts are biased by the three *gunas* (primal characteristics) and differ from person to person. To expound the works of Gorkashnath or say, the Buddha, is surely beyond the scope of their self-opinionated views. Their judgment is disturbed by thoughts. Only *samadhi* can experience *samadhi*. Only a Buddha can merge in Buddha. The scholar has reference books for crutches. The yogi flies free in search of his experiences and knows the suchness of things as they are.

You are a Soul and have a Body

People are not aware of their Soul. In general, they are unaware that they are a Soul because their consciousness has not been sufficiently integrated. It is spread out all over the body, in the seventy-two thousand motor sensory nerves. One has to, by yogic *pratyahara*, reverse the electrical flow of *prana* in the spinal cord. Subsequently one recollects and crystallizes one's Soul into what is called the *Jeevatma*.

The first stage is that the sincere disciple coalesces his Soul in the heart center as *Pranatma*. Then he, by further *sadhana* recollects his *mana* (his mind) into his Consciousness. He reverses the electric flow of *prana* and converts it into *Jeevatma*. Then, by further *pratyahara* and *sadhana* he goes into *dhyana* and *samadhi*. He transforms from *Pranatma* into *Jeevatma* and then from *Jeevatma* to *Paramatma* at the thousand-petal lotus. He has to practice the rightful yoga and make an effort to integrate the Soul within him.

Potentially, every man is a divine soul but he does not have the awareness. This is because his consciousness, in the form of *prana,* is spread all over his body. It is involved in the five senses. *Indra* (king of the gods) has fallen from his Soul throne in the third eye into the snares of his five *indriyas*, the queens of the senses, who are the cause of keeping many a Soul-*Indra* and yogi ensnared in sense distractions. By doing *Shiva-shakti Kriya Yoga*, he creates an electro-magnetic current in his spinal cord. This *kriya* is called the *mahatam janma aradhana*, meaning the most important *sadhana* in his life, whereby he crystallizes his Soul.

It is quite shocking that some people die senselessly as empty shells, where they cannot create the Soul-consciousness by this *sadhana* of *pratyahara*. You must withdraw your *pranic* energy from the five senses and recollect your Self-soul in your third eye. This is very important. That's why, when your own will is not used, as in drugs, the willpower becomes a pulp. And when your own will is not functioning and you are lazy, getting something easily, then you will be a helpless heap. Therefore, in so far as pure spirituality is concerned, where you recollect your bodily energy in the form of light in your third cyc, then that light (*tejas*) combines with love (*ojas*) and life (*prana*) to form the Conscious Soul in your third eye. This is most effectively done by a

yogic technique of *yoni mudra* which greatly assists in the evolution of consciousness. The Soul is seen as the third eye, a gold rim, blue center and white star.
Alakh Niranjan!

Guru-disciple Relationships

The first and foremost interaction between a teacher and the "to be taught," between a Master and a disciple, between a Guru and a *shishaya*, is the interaction of Divine love. How does this interaction of Divine love take place and what does it do? The interaction of Divine love takes place through the awakened *kundalini shakti* of the Guru to the receptive disciple in his navel *chakra*, the heart *chakra* and the third eye *chakra*.

And what does this transmission of love do? The main purpose of the transmission is the evolution of human Consciousness. It evolves human Consciousness from man the brute, to man the man, to man the God. This is where we are going, in spite of ourselves, because the warp and weft of the cosmic flow, the galactic swirl, is towards Divinity. And because the whole rhythm and music of the universe is towards Divinity, we cannot help but flow in that direction.

And the greatest servants of humanity are the gurus, the teachers of spiritual knowledge, the *Sat-Gurus*, the true ones who have their *kundalini* awakened and can give their disciples an evolutionary impetus. And the *Divya Gurus*, that is, the Divine Gurus who come from age to age like the Buddha, the Krishna, the Christ, they are the ones who have the power to evolve and transform whole humanities. The *Satguru* (a perfected Being in the work he is empowered to do) works upon his disciples with unconditional love. Like a sculptor, he sculpts out the marble stone of the disciple to make him into the beautiful Krishna, or the beautiful Christ. He gives of himself to make the disciple aware that every true Master will not only pray for himself and evolve his own Consciousness, but gives his life's blood and his energy to the disciples to enable them to evolve into the likeness of the indwelling Christ, the Goddess Durga, the likeness of the indwelling Krishna, or his Divine love Radha. The Master in his turn merges into his own divine indweller which in this case is Shiva Goraksha Babaji.

Appendix

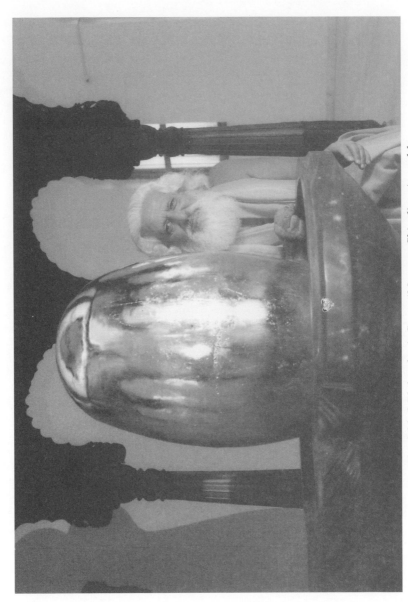

*The fabled Philsopher's Stone (Mercury Shivalinga) used by
Indian Nath Yogis for Kaya-Kalpa & Sanjeevani (Rejuvenation).*

ALCHEMICAL MERCURY SHIVALINGA
'A closely guarded mystery vortex'

At the convocation of Maha Shivaratri the Hamsa Yoga Sangh inaugurated the Earth Peace Temple at the Siddhanath Forest Ashram near Pune on the 6th of March 2008.

The Earth Peace Temple has been established to bring about unity and abiding peace amongst all peoples of the earth. "We teach no religion, people from all climes and times, races and religions are welcome with open arms".

The temple houses the world's largest solid (*akhand*) mercury Shivalinga. Mercury when purified and brought to a solid state is referred to as the elusive 'Philosopher's Stone' or 'Paras Mani' (the mercury gem). Meditating in the radiance of this Shivalinga rejuvenates and transforms the meditator. Its nectar-like-effects have been experienced by meditating Nath Yogis since time immemorial. **"The creation of this type of alchemical Mercury Shivalinga is a closely guarded secret of the Indan spiritual culture blessed by Shiva Gorarksha Babaji.** This rare Shivalinga is now ours to avail of and to use for the purpose of Earth Peace through Self Peace".

Over the past thirty years, along with my wife Shivangini we have with loving care in the gentle valley of Sita Mai, set up this powerful centre for spiritual seekers. Disciples and evolved souls from all over India and the world come to learn the evolutionary techniques of **Babaji's Kundalini Kriya Yoga**.

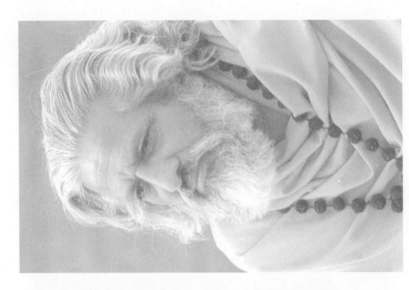

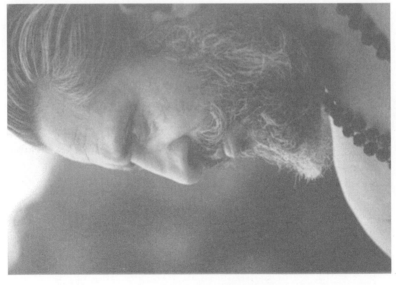

Yogiraj Siddhanath: The Yogi and The Spiritual Healer

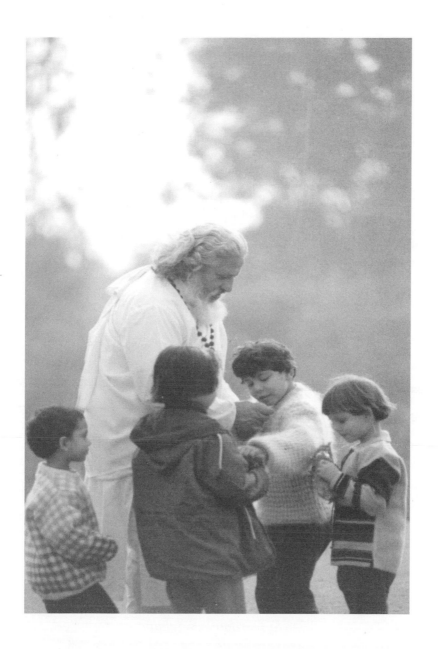

Yogiraj spreads his message of Love to the young

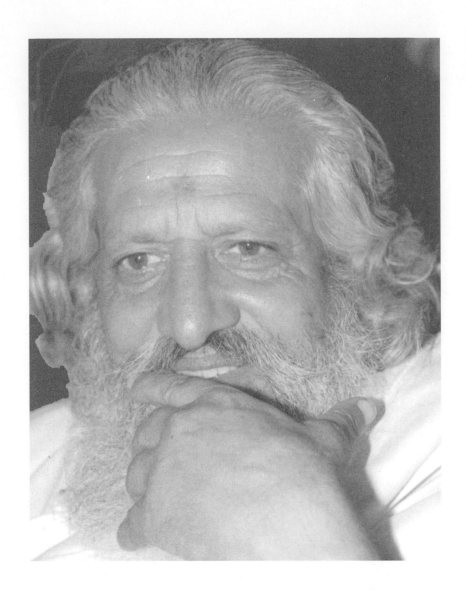

Yogiraj Gurunath Siddhanath

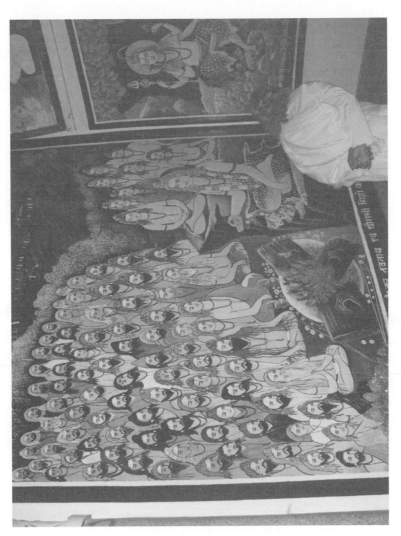

Siddhanath at Barthahari Cave, Haridwar

Shiva-Goraksha-Babaji

Who art Thou? I know Thee not
And yet I am of Thee
I cannot comprehend thee Lord,
Thou Emperor of Divinity

I sit and melt in silence of
Thy Love Oh Infinite
Make me thy Truth, Make me thy Love
Eternal Lord of Light

Countless creations do you make
Goraksha Nath Divine
A thought projected by you
Makes causation, space and time

There never was a Sage or Saint
Who was not born of Thee
Thou art the essence of their Souls
Divine Paramatma Free

We Jivatmas also Lord
Have our birth and being in Thee
Then Thou must also be in us
Supremest Monarchy

How shall I love Thee Babaji?
Words are so dry and dumb
I can't express Thy majesty
My intellect runs numb

My heart it bursts oh all in all
To love Thee endlessly
But Lord I cannot bring to words
I'm tongue-tied hopelessly

Give me the strength to shout Thy love
Across the seven seas
Deludging this world with light
For infinite eternities

In solitudes of my mind
My devotion it dost burst to hear
Thy song immortal song of love
Thou everlasting Seer

As long as darkness covers me
And ignorance doth do us part
So long in agony I'll be
Striving to be with Thee, my Heart

Through pain and hunger I shall strive
To touch Thy feet oh Lord
It matters not if bones or body
Perish in this battle fort

I'm burning in My love for Thee
Eternal Infinite
I cannot rest in peace now
Till I do become thy Light

In silent supplications
I do burn and yearn to be in Thee
Hear Thou my soul cry
Break my bonds, Babaji set me free

Set me free to be in Thee
Let there be none of me
Then me in Thee, Thy love in me
I shall become of Thee

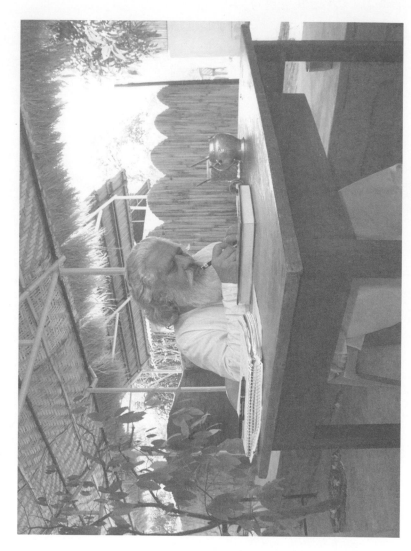

Writing at his forest ashram in Sinhagad

ON BEING A DISCIPLE OF BABAJI

YE SONS OF LIGHT DELUSION FIGHT
BE CONSTANT IN YOUR DAY AND NIGHT

It is my opinion that Babaji has taken no direct disciples after Yogavatar Lahiri Mahasaya, who had transformed his body into light, because only someone whose body is free from the ravages of time, in a perpetual state of *sahaj samadhi*, is fit for such a direct relationship.

It is one thing to have an experience of Babaji, but to be a DIRECT DISCIPLE of Babaji is quite a different echelon of realization. Many people have claimed to have experiences of the ineffable Babaji, but to be in a continuous state of a Guru-disciple electromagnetic rapport with Babaji (the Lord of Irradiant Splendor) is in my opinion an utterly impossible connection for mundane people. For the spiritual interaction between a human being and such a lofty phenomenon, would totally shatter the so-called disciple's body.

The nervous system, brain cells and *astral chakras* of a normal mortal being are not designed to capacitate the spiritual influx of such a cosmic Being like Mahavatar Babaji. Only an *avatar* is qualified to be a disciple of a *Mahavatar*. Any lesser being would merely be floating in the figment of one's own imagination. Because in reality, if cosmic lightning struck a mortal being, no matter however gently with the utmost of love, that mortal frame would vanish into nothing, unless by virtue of being an *Avataric* consciousness, like Buddha, Christ, Bharthari Nath, Chaurangi Nath and Lahiri Mahasaya, who can capacitate the voltage of the incoming Christos called Babaji.

Anyone claiming such a relationship would have to demonstrate the states of Lahiri Mahasaya or Sri Yukteswar, such as:
* *Shambhavey Mudra*: Unblinking outward gaze with inward

mind transformed to Soul-*samadhi*.

- *Nirvikalpa Samadhi*: In a state of divine conciousness beyond divine mind. Never sleeping, but always in *samadhi*.
- *Punarutthan:* Self-resurrection like Yogaavatar Lahiri Mahasaya, Gyanavatar Sri Yukteswar and Premavatar Jesus Christ.

When a person says he has a direct experience of Babaji, it is his word against the belief of the people. And there is no way to prove or disprove a truth or a lie. Only that person in his heart knows what he is saying, and Babaji metes out the final *karmic* justice.

Many people have had visions, visitations, blessings and guidance from this lofty Being. This is possible and this may be true. But so much is the spiritual difference between Babaji and mortal humans, that even a minimal spiritually-charged experience of such magnitude would leave the yogi in a daze for many days and months to come.

It must be remembered that when one claims to be a disciple of Babaji in the spiritual sense, his *kundalini* energy is ceaselessly connected with the *Cosmic Kundalini* of *Babaji*. And after the last case of Yogavatar Lahiri Mahasaya, I see no less a person being able to maintain a *Guru*-disciple relationship with this Cosmic Being. No doubt, they can be blessed or have visions, which are based on the painting of Babaji which was inspired by Yogananda's experience and hence those visions falls under the catagory of Savikalpa darshan. However to have the core experience of Babaji a Divine Being must go beyond the Dharmamegh Samadhi, the great rings pass not.

Over-enthusiastic practitioners and Swamis must guard against hallucinations or mistaking a three-dimensional vision as a certificate for being a direct disciple of Babaji—a sense of proportions is needed. There are many diseased and feeble *neophyte* devotees and Swamis who by the mere vision of Babaji have been cured of their ailments. This does not qualify them to be disciples of this *Cosmic Avatar but* graces them to march along their spiritual journey towards their final beatitude Babaji HimSelf.

It is sad but true that human nature has a tendency to "jump the fence," and wants to do the Ph.D. course before finishing kindergarten. To have a vision is okay, but to perpetually bathe in the cosmic aura of "a Being About Whom Naught May Be Said," is quite a different ball game. Although He is the divinity of the consciousness of the life of our breath closer to us then our very selves, let us truthfully introspect and be honest with ourselves as to where we stand in relation to Babaji. Our existence is his proof He is totally in us but how much of us have we realized in Him?

Babaji's entourage are very high initiates of the 8th degree, known as the Sages of the Fire Mist. Those are his disciples, if we can call them so; 33 in graded order, clothed in their glorious bodies, great beyond man's reckoning, their celestial forms'came to earth 18.5 million years ago to infuse the spirit of the Divine into the human phenomenon. As these are great Presences beyond the scope of birth and death when we say of them, He is dead! Behold He is alive! and appears somewhere else. These glorious beings never die for they were never born!

Here we must make a special mention of some lofty Sages of the Fire-mist who stand at the dizzying heights equal to the planetary and solar gods in the spiritual hirerarchy. The first is the Great Adi Guru Shankaracharya who was directed by Shiv Goraksha Babaji to infuse the highest science of *Advait* and spiritual evolution to thirsty humanity. The second of the lofty Beings is the great Dattatreya who also gave to this earth the philosophy of Advait and the mystic science of Tantra Yoga. There are others in his entourage who like the Gyanavatar Yukteshwar has been given the responsibility for evolving higher souls in the realms of Hiranyaloka (Golden Heaven). The Kalki Avatar or Maitreya Buddha are some of the lofty beings who are working in the cosmic aura of Babaji the King of Kings. The Kalki Avatar, who in the Christian Fraternity is called the Christ, is also called Maitreya who is getting ready to establish truth on earth.

The great Yogeshwari Umanath the consort of Shiva is also called Udaynath. She with her universal force personifies the cosmic kundalini and is also working at the eighth level with Sages of the Fire-mist in assisting the evolution of human consciousness to attain the final realization. From her is projected to the seventh Avataric level the divine feminine energy of the World Mothers (Regina Munde) whose sacred womb served as the divine receptacle in Kausalya the mother of Ram, Devki the mother of Krishna, Maya the mother of Buddha and Mary the mother of Christ and so also is the case when the great Kalki avatar incarnates at the dawn of the leo-aquarius age.

There are other beings who are in Babajis Entourage who form the spiritual hierarchy of our world in finely graded order. They are blessed, and are *Avatars* and Buddhas and Manus. Here are some of their names: Lord Maitreya, who is Christ, who is to come as the Kalki Avatar, our world Saviour and Teacher. Lord Vaivashvat Manu Spiritual King of our world, then King Vikramaditya (El Morya) who is to succeed the Manu. King Devapi (Kuthumi), who is to succeed Lord Kalki as the next world Teacher. Then we come to some of Chiranjeevs meaning Immortals Lord Hanuman, Ashvathama, Karna, Arjuna, Nagarjun, Aaryasangh, Count St.Germain, Parshurama, Bali, Kashayap, Lord Surya (our Sun) who is one of the most glorious and venerated Sages of fire-mist who works along with Shiv Goraksha Babaji. So high is His spiritual stature that there are very few words to say.

Of course, let me add that there are other Babajis about whom people have written. Some are mortal, some are true historical beings, and some are totally fictitious. These "babajis" go by various names. About these babajis and their disciples and followers, I have nothing to say, since any elderly person can call himself babaji, meaning "revered father", and claim to have had a direct vision and even build a temple in his name.

Now I would caution the western world about the true "Babaji" and not be led into believing a figment of their imagination. To be on solid ground, look for authentic historical evidences of temples, books and other literature, which are ancient documents written about this wondrous Being. Because, other wondrous beings, like the Lord Krishna and the Lord Christ, also appeared to people on earth and told them where they were born, and where they were crucified. The vestiges and traces of their historical episodes are still on earth today. Then surely temples and books by, of, and about the great Babaji, must be around. LOOK! For such an immortal being we are left with a glaring Truth that Babaji Gorakshanath, or Shiva-Goraksha-Babaji, is the one and only living example of this Lord of Irradiant Splendor, with temples and historical evidences throughout the length and breadth of the land of India. It is about this Supernal Being that I am talking, and to whom I am referring.

Glossary

A

abhyas: 'perservering practice', a practice which brings about disspassion (*vairagya*) and discernment (*vivek*).

acharya: a preceptor, instructor, or teacher-guru.

adharma: all that is contrary to the law and what is right.

Adinath: 'Primordial Lord', the founder of the *Nath Yogis*, Shiva Himself

Advaita: 'nonduality', the truth and teaching that there is only One Reality called *Atman or Brahman*, especially as found in the *Upanishads*; *see also Vedanta*

agni: presiding deity of the element of fire.

agya chakra: 'command center', a yogic appellation for the third eye center; center of Divine Presence located at the midpoint between the eyebrows; *see kutastha chaitanya*

ahamkara: 'I-maker', the individuation principle, or ego, which must be transcended; *see also asmita, buddhi, manas.*

Ahirbudnya: 'Unfathomable Serpent of the Deep', epithet of Lord Shiva.

ahimsa: 'non-harming', an important moral discipline (*yama*).

aja: 'the unborn', a term used for the primordial Divine as well as its universal energy called *Kundalini*.

aja ekapada: 'the unborn one-footed', also translated as, 'he who stands alone on one leg, without support.'

akarma: 'actionless action', karmaless action

Akasha: 'Radiant Æther', 'Deva Bramanaspati' also personified in Greece as 'Zeus'. The homogenious fabric of luminosity composing the physical universe; the first of the five cosmic elements designates inner-space, that is, the space of Consciousness (*cid-akasha*).

Akashic records : All thought forms & deeds of past, present & future called the 'Triform Karma' of humanity is impressed as records in this homogenious fabric of radient æther

Akula: 'nonflock', an epithet of Lord Shiva.

Alakh Niranjana: 'The Lightless Light which lights that light which lights the light in all our soul'; a name for God and a greeting, voiced by *Nath Yogis.*

Amanaska Yoga: 'the Yoga beyond mind', a work on hatha yoga ascribed to Gorakshanath. It is a technique for the simultaneous stabilization of one's gaze, breathing and attention which brings about a no-mind state; *see unmani avasta.*

Amba: 'Great Deep', appellation for an aspect of the Divine Mother.

amrita: 'immortal', a designation of the deathless Soul (*atma-purusha*); the nectar of immortality that flows from the psycho-energetic center at the crown of the head (*sahasrara-chakra*) when it is activated by yogic means, transforming the physical body into a divine body (*divya-deha*).

anahata chakra: 'wheel of the unstruck sound', the twelve-petal lotus of the heart. The heart has since ancient times been viewed as the secret seat of Vasudeva and the location where the immortal sound *Om* can be heard. Its seed syllable (*bija mantra*) is *yam* pertaining to the element of wind.

ananda: 'bliss', the condition of utter joy, which is an essential quality of the ultimate reality (*tattva*) described as *sat-chit-ananda*.

Ananda Kanda: 'seat of joy', situated low within the anahat chakra with eight petals; the seat of Krishna Vasudev (the 'shining-one residing in the heart') holding the passport to paradise for all transmigrating souls   It is located within the causal body, the *anandamayeekosha* (*ananda-maya-kosha*).

anga: 'limb', a fundamental category of the yogic path, such as *yama*, *niyama*, *asana*, *pranayama*, *pratyahara*, *dharana*, *dhyana*, *samadhi*

annamaya-kosha: 'sheath composed of food', the lowest of the five 'envelopes' (*kosha*) covering the Self; the physical body

apana: the downward flowing life-force energy in the spine. In *Kriya Yoga* it is used for dissolving *karma*

apas: 'water'.

aranyaka: 'that which pertains to the forest', an early type of ritual text used by forest-dwelling sages; *see also Upanishad.*

arbandha-nag langot: the wollen belts tied around the waist of the *Nath Yogi* extending to form a part of his under-garment; also calld the *bhairava bana*

arti: the waving & blessing of the light and sound during divine worship

Arjuna: 'fair', one of the five *Pandava* princes who fought in the *Mahabharata War*; disciple of the *Avatar Krsna* whose teachings can be found in the *Bhagavad-Gita.*

asana: 'seat', a physical posture (see also *anga, mudra*); the third limb (*anga*) of *Patanjali's* eightfold path (*asthanga-yoga*); originally this meant only meditation posture, but subsequently, in *Hatha Yoga*, this aspect of the yogic path was developed further; *also* the seat upon which a yogi sits durng meditation.

ashram: a vanaprastha hermitage (forest dweller); third stage of life, such as *brahmacharya* is first, householder - second, and complete renunciate - final stage (*samnyasin*), 'where nishkam karma is done', the devotee works without desire for reward creating no new karma.

astral chakras: the chakras corresponding to the astral body.

Ashtanga Yoga: 'eight-limbed union', the eightfold Yoga of Patanjali, consisting of moral discipline (*yama*), self-restraint (*niyama*), posture (*asana*), breath control (*pranayama*), sensory withdrawal (*pratyahara*), concentration (*dharana*), meditation (*dhyana*), and ecstasy (*samadhi*), leading to liberation (*kaivalya*).

asmita: 'I-am-ness', concept of the ego in Patanjali's eight-limbed Yoga, *see ahamkara.*

atman: 'self', the true Self, the individual spirit or soul, which is eternal and super-conscious; our true nature or identity; sometimes a distinction is made between the *atman* as the individual self and the *parama-atman* as the transcendental Self; *see also purusha, brahman*

aunsch avatara: A partial *avatara* that manifests only the degree of Divinity necessary to fulfill a specific mission.

aulia: 'The Divine Madman', a God-intoxicated yogi between the 3rd and 6th degree initiation; *see mast.*

avadhoot: 'cast-off', he who has shed everything; a *Nath Yogi* who having gone through the 6th stage of initiation, by both his individual effort and Divine grace, achieved the Consciousness of the *avatar.*

avasta: 'condition', the super-conscious states of Yoga distinguished according to the level of refinement of God Realization.

avatar: 'descent', the descent of the Divine into a terrestrial light-body for spiritual work and the salvation of the world; identified outwardly by specific signs, such as the tendency of the *avatar* to cast no shadow.

Avatars of Vishnu: incarnations of Lord Vishnu, each with a specific purpose.

avidya: 'ignorance', the root cause of suffering (*duhkha*); also called *ajnana;* cf. *vidya*

Ayurveda: 'the science of longevity', one of India's traditional systems of medicine employing the use of herbs, foods, and metals. The eldest of the world's medical systems.

B

Babaji: 'Revered father', in the *Nath* tradition, the name denoting Shiva Goraksha Babaji; 'The Youth of 16 Summers'; 'The Ever-Youthful Immortal Yogi'; also mentioned in Yogananda's book, *Autobiography of a Yogi.*

banda: 'seal' or 'lock', a constriction of certain muscles in the *Hatha* and *Kriya Yoga* systems for locking in *prana* and ushering *kundalini* energy up the *sushumna-nadi* of the spine.

beedi: rolled up dry tobacco leaf used for smoking.

Bhagavad-Gita: 'Lord's Song', the most popular book on the science of Yoga, embedded in the epic *Mahabharata* and containing the teachings of *Karma Yoga* (the path of self-transcending action), *Jnana Yoga* (the path of wisdom), *Bhakti Yoga* (the path of devotion), and *Raja Yoga* (the supreme path of meditation) as given by the Avatar Krsna to Prince Arjuna on the battlefield of Kurushetra

bhajan: from the root *bhaj* 'to divide', devotional song whence the devotee is separate from Deity and does not fuse with God as does the yogi in *samadhi*

bhakta: 'devotee', a disciple practicing *Bhakti Yoga*

bhakti: 'devotion' or 'love', the love of the *bhakta* toward the Divine or the Guru as a manifestation of the Divine

Bhakti Sutra: 'Aphorism of Devotion', an aphoristic work on devotional Yoga authored by Sage *Narada* given by Lord Shiva.

Bhakti Yoga: 'Yoga of devotion', a major branch of the Yoga tradition utilizing the feeling capacity to connect with the ultimate reality conceived of as a personal Divinity.

Bharat: the land whose people are wedded to the light of the Soul; the land of India

Bhavani: the feminine aspect of Shiva dwelling in the seven heavens (*bhavanas*) of *Bhur, Bhuva, Svaha, Maha, Jana, Tapah,* and *Satya* (seventh heaven).

bhuta: 'to become', the material elements, also called *pancha bhuta*, or five elements of earth (*prithvi*), water (*apas*), fire (*agni*), air (*vata*), and space (*akasha*)

bhuta shuddhi: 'purification of the elements', transformation of the gross physical body into a Divine body, by dissolving the five elements

bija-mantra: (*Beej-mantra*) 'seed word', a monosyllabic *mantra*, each of which is associated with one of the seven *chakras* of the body

bindu: 'seed-point', the creative potency of anything where all energies are focused; the red dot worn on the forehead as indicative of the third eye.

bodhi: 'enlightenment', the state of the awakened Master, or Buddha.

bodhisattva: 'enlightened being', the *Chiranjiv* immortals and *avadhoots* whose bodhi-chitta (*buddhi*) are purfied to such a degree of compassion that they spurn Nirvana (*moksha*) to serve humanity.

Brahma: 'he who has grown expansive', the creator of the universe, the first principle (*tattva*) to emerge out of the ultimate reality (*brahman*).

brahma gufa: see *Cave of Brahma*

Brahma Nirvana: merging in the transcendental core beyond the universe. Being everywhere and nowhere at the same time Kaivalya.

brahmacharya: the discipline of chastity for the channelisation of vital energy (*prana*) and trnsformation into *ojas* and *tejas* by the practice of *Shiva-Shakti Kriya Yoga* and *Mahamudra*.

Brahman: 'that which has grown expansive', the ultimate reality cf. *atman, purusha*)

Buddha: 'awakened', a designation of the person who has attained enlightenment (*bodhi*) and therefore inner freedom; term designating *Gautama*, the founder of Buddhism, who lived in the sixth centuryBCE

buddhi: 'that which is conscious, awake', the higher mind, which is the seat of wisdom (*jnana*); *manas*.

C

Cave of Brahma: '*Brahma Gumfa*', the brain's third ventricle; a hollow space in the human brain formed by the thalimus as its walls, the hypothalimus as its floor, and the third choroid plexus as its roof

chakra: '*pranic* wheel', the psycho-energetic centers of the subtle body (*sukshma-sharir*). Classically seven of such centers are given: *muladhara chakra* at the perineum, *svadhishthana chakra* at the base of the spine, *manipura chakra* at the navel, *anahata chakra* at the heart, *vishuddhi chakra* at the throat, *ajna chakra* in the middle of the head, and *sahasrara chakra* at the top of the head.

Chandogya Upanishad: one of the oldest scriptures written in 200 BCE; it's contents elaborate on the nature of *Om* and *prana*.

Chauhan: Lord

Chiranjeev: 'Immortals', at the level of avadhoot and above, whose body-mind is purified to such a degree of compassion that they spurn *Nirvana Moksha* to serve humanity as their Larger Self; *see also Bodhisattva*.

Chrestos: is the high initiate traveling from the 5th to the 6th degree of initiation, representing the vibrition in relativity; the Holy Spirit.

Christ: the 7th degree initiate; the World Teacher; an *avatar* such as Kalki Avatar, Maitreya, Matsyendranath, Avalokiteshwara, Vithoba (the man crucified in space).

Christos: the Divine higher-Self called Archangel Michael, Narayan 'the Lord of Irradiant Splendor', and Amitabh. The Christos has crossed the 8th degree of the great initiations. Above them there is only one, 'The Eternal Now,' Shiv-Goraksha Babaji.

cit: 'consciousness', the super-conscious ultimate reality (see *Atman, Brahman,Chaitanya*)

citta: 'mind-substance', ordinary consciousness, the mind, as opposed to *cit*.

citi: '*shakti*', kinetic energy; *see kundalini*.

connectus conarsus: common connecting factor between the whole of humanity, the breath, pran & sutratma, (the thread soul which flows through humanity).

Cosmic Kundalini: the universal life force and light which gives birth to subsequent Creation.

D

dakini: 'a sky-walker', a semi-divine female being, sometimes progressing one's spiritual practice and sometimes obstructing it.

darshana: 'Insight', divine vision; receiving of blessings from a Divine Guru or spiritual Being; or of a system of philosophy, such as the *yoga-darshana* of *Patanjali*

Deva: 'shining one', a male deity, such as Shiva, Vishnu, or Brahma, either in the sense of the ultimate reality (*Maha Deva*) or a high angelic being.

Deva Rishi: Rishi, Raj Rishi, Dev Rishi & Bramha Rishi, third in the hierarchical order of *Rishis*.

Devi: 'shining one', the feminine aspect of *deva*; a goddess or feminine angelic being such as Parvati, Lakshmi, or Saraswati.

dhaba: a place of roadside fast-food in India

dharana: 'holding', concentration, the sixth limb (*anga*) of Patanjali's eight-limbed (*ashtanga*) system of Yoga.

dharma: 'bearer', law or lawfulness, also correct action, conduct and righteousness and vitue.

Dharma megha samadhi: '*samadhi* of the Cloud of Forms', it is neither the cloud nor the forms but the actual showering of enlightenment as the cloud drifts away; and the sun of God Realization is experienced, then the *yogeshwar* is merged in the absolute called *Kaivalya*.

dhuni: the sacred fires of the ancient yogis revered as holy and sustaining their livlihood for cooking and warmth and alkaline cow dung ash (*gow-rakh*) used to prevent disease and maintain body temperature in both hot and cold conditions.

dhyana: meditation; seventh limb (*anga*) of Patanjali's eight-limbed Yoga brought about as a result of correct concentration (*dharana*); later called *cha'an* by the Chinese and rendered still later as *zen* by the Japanese .

diksha: 'initiation', the act and condition of induction into the hidden aspects of Yoga or a particular lineage of teachers; all traditional Yoga involves *diksha* from a Master.

divya-deha: 'divine body', a divine body of radiant light created by yogic ingestion of mercury, pranayama, diet, and God's grace. An immaculate body of rainbow light, free from the ravages of time for the purpose of uninterrupted communion with God; *see also divya-vapus.*

Divya Guru: 'Divine preceptor', a Guru who works from a higher plane of existence, astral or causal.

duhkha: 'bad axle space', suffering; the condition of mortality caused by ignorance (*avidya*) of our divine nature (*atman*).

Durga: The cardinal goddess of Hinduism, spouse of Lord Shiva.

dvesha: hatred, aversion

E

Elohim: a name of God in the Hebrew tradition; also the heavenly host of gods and angels in the Hebrew tradition.

F

feng shui: the science of Geomancy **derived from the ancient** *Vastu Shastra* **of India**, originated by the being Vastuspati, Lord Shiva, who gave it to Vishvakarma, the architecht of the celestials and the universe. *Vastu gyan* later spread to China & was called *Feng Shui.*

G

Gabastiman: 'Lord of Irradiant Splendor', name of the Spiritual Sun.

gandha: one of the principle conduits of prana; pertaining to smell.

Gayatri Mantra: a Vedic *mantra* recited to enlighten the intellect and give liberation (*moksha*) chanted at the junctions of sunrise and sunset (*sandhikal*).

ghagara-chunari: a style of *Rajasthani* dress and Northern India including a tunic, top, and shawl.

Ghandarva: race of celestial beings specializing in music.

ghat: a small temple in Banares along the holy river Ganges for worship and bathing rituals.

Gheranda Samhita: The Master Gheranda's compendium on *Hatha Yoga*, consisting of 351 stanzas and presented as a dialogue between Gheranda and his disciple Candakapali. This work is modeled on the earlier work, the *Hatha Yoga Pradikipa* 'light on the Sun/Moon Yoga' authored by Svatmarama Yogi with the contents of Shiv-Goraksha Babaji.

Godessence: a word coined by Yogiraj Siddhanath which includes God and Goddess as the highest spiritual essence possible in the domain of Relativity; beyond that is the ineffable state of the Non-being Essentiality.

God-Realization: "Those who tell it know it not and those who know it tell it not." says Yogiraj Siddhanath.

Goraknathi: a devotee or follower of Goraknath; also called a *Kanphat Yogi* or *Gorakh Panthi*.

Goraksha: *see Gorakshanath*

Gorakshanath: 'Lord Goraksha', Babaji; also called Shiva-Goraksha-Babaji, a renownly well documented *avatar* of Indian Yogic tradition, responsble for hastening the spiritual evolution of humanity. The personal aspect of Lord Shiva. *see also Mahavtar.*

goshti: spiritual chat from a Guru.

gotra: a spiritual lineage

Gotrabhu: 'matured and ready', for the next higher initiation.

granthi: 'knot', any one of three common blockages in the central pathway (*sushumna-nadi*) preventing the full ascent of the serpent power (*kundalini-shakti*); the three knots are known as *Brahma granthi* (at the *muladhara chakra*), the *Vishnu granthi* (at the heart), and the *Rudra granthi* (at the third-eye center).

Guardian Wall of Humanity: is composed of high initiates called the Siddhas of the 5th degree.They protect our fragile humanity from harms way. *see Siddha Sangh.*

guna: 'quality', refers to any of the three primary 'qualities' or constituents of nature (*prakriti*): *tamas* (the principle of inertia), *rajas* (the dynamic principle), and *sattva* (the principle of lucidity)

guru: 'one with gravity', a teacher who cultivates the spiritual knowledge of a disciple.

guru bhakti: a disciple's self-transcending devotion to his or her guru.

Guru Dabar: conclave of spiritual monarchs

Guru Yoga: a spiritual discipline found in the tradition of Yoga whereby the Guru becomes the center of a disciple's practice.

gyan: *see jnana.*

Gyan Swaroop: embodiment of wisdom.

H

Hamsa: 'swan', the Soul, the individuated Consciousness (*jiva*); also refers to the life-breath (*prana*) as it moves within the body; the lateral ventricles in the human brain in the shape of a swan in flight, with its wings thrust toward the forehead and its posterior ventricle pointed to the back, like a swan flying back to the future, faster than light; *see jiva-atman.*

Hamsa Kriyacharya: a teacher of the 3rd level of initiation; not to be confused with the more advanced Hamsanath Yogi of the Great Initiations.

Hamsa Yoga: 'swan yoga'; ancient text in the form of a conversation between Sanatana Kumar (an important aspect of Shiv Goraksha Babaji), and his pupil Gautama; this is Kundalini Kriya Yoga, giving the levels of manifestions of the resonance of *Omkar.*

Hamsa Yogi: practioner of Hamsa Yoga.

Hamsacharya: a teacher of the *Hamsa Yoga Sangh* at the 2nd level of initiation.

Hamsanet: the astral light connection formed by Yogiraj Satgurunath connecting all of the disciples (*Hamsas*) to the Satguru and to one another.

Haribol: 'say Hari', one of the many names of Lord Vishnu

Hatha Yoga: 'Forceful Yoga', a major branch of Yoga, developed by Gorakshanath, emphasizing the physical aspects of the transformative path, notably postures (*asana*) and cleansing techniques (*shodhana*), but chiefly breath control (*pranayama*) leading right upto samadhi.

Hatha Yoga Pradikipa: a branch of Yogic knowledge given by Shiva-Goraksha Babaji, 'light on the Sun/Moon Yoga' compiled by Svatmarama Yogi. This work comprises 389 couplets, and integrates the practices of Hatha and Raj Yoga.

Hiranyaloka: 'golden world', the highest astral heaven of luminosity to which some yogis ascend, to practice higher forms of Yoga (e.g. Nirvikalpa Samadhi)under the guidance of Divine Teachers such as Shri Yukteswar

I

Iccha Shakti: 'will-power', the first of three aspects of divine power, the other two being *Gyan Shakti* 'knowledge power,' and *Kriya Shakti*, 'creative power.'

ida nadi: 'pale conduit', the *prana* current or arc ascending on the left side of the central channel (*sushumna-nadi*) associated with the parasympathetic nervous system and having a cooling or calming effect on the mind when activated; cf. *pingala-nadi*

indriya: 'concerning Indra', the five senses of sight, hearing, taste, smell, touch, and the corresponding organs of sense.

Is-ness of the Zero-not-Zero: Yogiraj has coined this term. The zero represents the Nothing of Creation. The naught-zero represents the Everything in Creation and the Is-ness pervades them and is beyond them both.

Ishta Devata: the principal aspect of God according to one's devotion

Ishvara: 'ruler', the Lord; an epithet or reference to God such as the Creator (Brahma) or, in Patanjali's *Yoga-Darshana*, to a special transcendental Self (*purusha*)

Ishvara-pranidhana: offering one self to the Lord & Guru as the priority; in Patanjali's eight-limbed Yoga one of the practices of Kriya Yoga. The other two being Tapah & Swadhyaya.

Ishwara-Sanatana: 'God Eternal', the *Mahavatara*, Shiva-Goraksha-Babaji.

J

Jagat: 'the world of change in a constant of flux called creation (samsara)'.

Jain: from *jinas* 'conquerors', the liberated adepts of Jainism; a member of Jainism, the spiritual tradition founded by Mahavira, a contemporary of Gautama the Buddha

japa: 'recitation', the repeated recitation of *mantras* to focus and clarify one's mind for meditation.

jiva: 'individual self', the individuated consciousness, as opposed to the ultimate Self (*param atman*); *also jivatman*

jivanmukta: an adept who, while still embodied, has attained liberation (*moksha*) from his material condtion (*samsara*).

jivanmukti: 'living liberation', the state of liberation while embodied

jnana: 'knowledge' or 'wisdom', both worldly knowledge or world-transcending wisdom, depending on the context; *also gyan*; *see also prajna, vidya*

Jnana Yoga: 'Yoga of wisdom', the path to liberation based on wisdom, or the direct intuition of the transcendental Self (*atman*) through the steady application of discernment between the real and the unreal, the Self and the not-self and renunciation of what has been identified as unreal or inconsequential to the achievement of liberation.

Jwala Kula: 'flame of the yogic family', an *avadhoot* now in a Tibetan body. In his former life he was Aaryasangh, the great exponent of the *Yogachara School* of *Taraka Raj Yoga*.

K

karmasakshi: 'witness to the deeds of mortals', referring here to the sun incarnated as Lord Ram, a solar Avatar.

Kaivalya: 'isolation', the state of absolute freedom from conditioned existence, as explained in *Ashtanga Yoga*; in the non-dualistic traditions of India, this is usually called *moksha* or *mukti*, 'release' from the fetters of ignorance (*avidya*), total enlightenment in Aloneness !

Kal: 'Time', the duration between one event and another.

kala chakra: 'wheel of time'

Kali: a Goddess embodying the fierce (dissolving) aspect of the Divine

Kali Yuga: in the Hindu astralogical system, the dark age of spiritual and moral decline; the current god age of the world in the universal cycle, not to be confused with the shorter human age equinoctial cycle expounded by Sri Yukteswar.

Kalki/Maitreya: the coming of the 10th *Avatar* of Lord Vishnu.

Kalki Purana: an ancient treatise about the coming of the Kalki Avatar/ Maitreya who shall restore spirituality on this earth, and reinstate the Solar & Lunar Dynasties of righteousness.

kalpa: the lifespan assigned to our planetary system.

kama: 'desire', the appetite for sensual pleasure leading to the fulfillment of past life desires then sublimation and then to liberation (mokshya).

Kapila: the sage founder of the *Samkhya* tradition and composer of the *Samkhya Sutra.*

kara hati: 'to do with the hands', a form of martial arts originated in India known contemporarily as Karate.

karma: 'action', activity of any kind, including ritual acts; the law of cause and effect, of balance and justice, binding one to material condition; destiny; the condition of an individual birth.

Karma Yoga: 'Yoga of action', the liberating path of self-transcending action invovlving virtuous deeds (*punya*), holy ritual (*puja*), and astralogically prescribed methods.

kamandalu: a pot made of copper and brass and used by yogis for carrying water.

karuna: 'compassion', universal empathy complementary to wisdom (*prajna*) and essential to the path of liberation (Yoga).

Kaulism: *also Kaula-marga*, The *Kaul Tantra* originated by Matsyendranatha as disclosed in the Kaula-Jnana-Nirnaya involving the divinization of the body through stimulating the flow of 'the nectar of immortality' (*amrit*).

kaya kalpa: the Yogic Science of bodily rejuvenation and life extension for the purpose of prolonging one's meditation on God, originated by the *Nath Yogis.*

kevali samadhi: 'condition of aloneness', he who has 'become alone' and is established in seeing the Self.

khayal: Intutive musings

khechari mudra: 'space-walking seal'; facilitates astral travel. The yogic practice of 'swallowing the tongue' in order to seal the life energy (*prana*) to be given by a bonified Guru; the seal of the tongue beyond the ulvula, stimulating the pituitary gland to drink of *amrit*).

kosha: 'casing', any one of five 'envelopes' surrounding the transcendental Self (*atman*) and blocking its realization of its Divine nature: *annamayakosha* 'envelope made of food,' the physical body, *pranamayakosha* 'envelope made of life force,' *manomaya-kosha* 'envelope made of mind,' *vijnanamaya-kosha* 'envelope made of consciousness,' and *anandamayakosha* 'envelope made of bliss.'

Krshna: an incarnation (*Purna avatar*) of the God Vishnu, his teachings are in the *Bhagavad-Gita* and *Bhagavata-Purana*. Lived 3102 BCE

krittika: The **constellation pleiades,** the six star wives of the seven star sages of the Great Bear. The 7th wife Arundhati is with her Lord Vashishtha, the penultimate star of the constilation of the Great Bear also called Ursa Major

Kriya Yoga: 'Yoga of doing', the 'lightning path' which brings you to the path of non-doing (*akarma*); given by Babaji Gorakshanath for the dissolution of *karma* and acceleration of human evolution to Divinity.

kumbhaka: 'potlike', in the science of Yoga, the retention of the breath and constriction of the locks (*bandas*) to usher vital energy (*prana*) into the spinal cord (*sushumna nadi*) for the awakening of *kundalini*; *see also puraka, recaka*

kundalini: 'coiled serpant of the fire-kundh', electro-magnetic *pranic* energy centralized in the spine; *Kundalini* is the lady of the cinders whom, when fanned by the alchemical fire of *Shiva-Shakti pranayam*, ignites and blazes up the chimney of the spine to unite with the immortal Lord Shiva in the crown *chakra* (*sahasrara*) to enlighten the yogi.

Kundalini Kriya Yoga: *Kriya Yoga*; when the *Kriya Yoga pranayam* is performed, the *pranic* life-force in one's spinal chord (*sushumna*) builds up to generate a great spiritual magnetism and voltage. By the ceaseless movement of the *Shiva-Shakti Kriya*, life-force (*prana*), breath, vital fluid, and mind become one to form the evolutionary life-force energy called *Kundalini*.

kutastha chaitanya: Living light of the soul (*jeevatma*) in *agya chakra*

L

Lakulish: 'the staff-holder', 'He who holds the lightning-staff of evolution', a representation of Lord Shiva or Babaji-Gorakhnath; also deified as the ancient founder of the *Shiva Pashupat* sect of yogis.

lateral ventricles: the hollow lateral spaces of the human brain filled with cerebral spinal fluid; when the consciousness of a yogi fills the lateral ventricles, he sees the hollow space in the form of a swan in flight with its wings thrust towards the forehead and its head pointing to the back as though the Soul Swan is flying back to the future faster than light; *see Hamsa Swan*

Laya Yoga: 'Yoga of dissolution', an advanced form or process of *Tantric Yoga* by which the energies associated with the various psycho-energetic centers (*chakras*) of the subtle body are gradually dissolved through the ascent of the serpent power (*kundalini shakti*)

Linga: 'mark', the pillar of light as the creative principle; a symbol and popular icon of Lord Shiva; a symbol of the Everywhere & the Nowhere.

linga sharir: the subtle or psychic body that becomes more active during the dream state, the three sheaths of intelligence, mind and vital energy constitute this body.

lungi: a type of wraparound worn by the men of India

M

Maha Raja: great king

Mahabharata: 'Great Bharata', one of two of India's ancient and famous epics during the time of Lord Krishna, telling of the great war between the Pandavas and the Kauravas and serving as a repository for many spiritual and moral teachings.

Mahabhinishkar: 'the Great Sacrifice', the author refers to Shiv-Goraksha Babaji, the highest Be-ness of Divinity, who explodes himself to enter the atoms of all sentient and non-sentient beings and evolve humanity and creation to Divinity. **This Divinity gives completely of itsef and yet remains complete.** This divine enigma is beyond the scope of our humanity and gods to understand.

Mahan Kal: 'The Great Beyond Time', epithet of Lord Shiva.

Mahatma: 'great self', 'a great soul;' an honorific title bestowed on particularly meritorious individuals, such as Gandhi.

Mahishasur Mardini: an aspect of the warrior goddess Durga, 'slayer of the demon Mahishasur'.

manas: 'mind', the lower mind, which is bound to the senses and yields information (*vijnana*) rather than wisdom (*jnana, vidya*); cf. *buddhi*

mandala: 'circle', a circular design symbolizing the cosmos and specific to a deity. A protective aura of energy such as the *Nath Mandala*.

mantra: from the root *man* 'to think', a sacred sound or phrase, such as *om*, *hum*, or *om namah shivaya*, that has a transformative effect on the mind of the individual reciting it; to be ultimately effective, a *mantra* needs to be given in an initiation by a Master.

Mantra Yoga: the yogic path utilizing *mantras* as the primary means of liberation.

Manu: the primordial father of the human race.

Manu Savarni: El Morya Vikramaditya who is to succeed Spiritual King Vaivasvat Manu as the 8th future Manu.

marman: 'meridian centre', in Yoga and *Ayurveda*, a vital spot on the physical body where energy is concentrated or blocked; cf. *granthi* & *lethal spot*.

Matsyendranath: 'Fish Lord', an early *Nath* and *Mahasiddha*, who founded the *Yogini-Kaula* school of *Tantra* and who implored Shiva to give him a disciple more advanced than himself; the Guru of Gorakshanath on the earthly plane and his disciple in the celestial plane.

maya: 'measure', the deluding or illusive power of the world binding one to mortality; illusion by which the world is seen as separate from the Divine; ignorance, specifically in the form of duality.

Moksha: 'liberation', the condition of freedom from ignorance (*avidya*) and the binding effect of *karma*; also called *mukti, Kaivalya*

morchal: a fan made of peacock feathers used by the Guru for cleansing one's astral body and driving away negative forces.

Mrityu Loka: the world of mortals, the land where death is inevitable. Yama the god of death, it is said was the first mortal to die.

mudra: 'seal', a hand gesture (such as *chin mudra*) or whole-body gesture (such as *Mahamudra*) performed for the flow of subtle energies.

mula-mantra: 'root mantra', the root *mantra* of a specific deity; in the case of Shiva, *Om Namah Sivaya*; in the case of Visnu, *Om Namo Bagavate Vasudevaya*

muni: 'silent', a sage who has taken a vowel not to speak, to accumulate the energy of speech (*vac*) for the awakening of *Kundalini*.

N

nada: 'sound', the inner sound of *Om*, as it can be heard through the practice of *Nada Yoga*; *see also Hamsa Yoga*.

Nada Yoga: Yoga of the inner sound; the Yogic practice or process of producing and intently listening to the inner sound as a means of concentration and ecstatic self-transcendence

nadi: 'conduit', one of 72,000 subtle-astral channels along or through which the life force (*prana*) circulates; the three most prominant being the *ida nadi, pingala nadi*, and *sushumna nadi*.

nadi-shodhana: 'channel cleansing', the practice of purifying the conduits (nadies) for higher evolutionary states of Yoga, especially by means of life energy control (*pranayama*).

Naga: serpent beings who act as agents of weather phenomenon also called the Dragons of wisdom.

Narada: a Deva Rishi and devotee of Shiva who taught him divine music at Rudraprayag. He is the author of the *Bhakti-Sutras* as given by Lord Shiva.

Nath: 'Lord', appellation for the Masters of Yoga, the Lords of all forms of Yoga; orders of the maha siddhas founded by Gorakshanath also called chohans in Theosophical literature on mahatmas.

Nath Mandala: The electromagnetic spiritual field of the *Nath Yogis*

Nava-Nath: The primeval *Nine Naths* who have gone beyond the seventh degree of cosmic consciousness.

neophyte: a newly initiate pupil on the path; as he treads the path he is called a tenderfoot.

niranjana: a term used by *Nath Yogis* for the highest state of consciousness (s*amadhi*). The lightless light of *Kaivalya*.

nirbeeja: consciousness without seed; the highest form of *samadhi* before the *dharma megha samadhi* & final dissolution into *Kaivalya*.

nirodha: 'restriction', in Patanjali's eight-limbed Yoga, the very basis of the process of concentration, meditation, and ecstasy; in the first instance, the restriction of the 'whirls of the mind' (*chitta-vritti*).

Nirvana: cessation of all desire. synonymous with enlightenment; *see also Kaivalya*.

Nirvana Moksha: *see Brahma Nirvana, Kaivalya*

niyama: 'self-restraint', the second limb of Patanjali's eightfold path, which consists of purity (*shauca*), contentment (*samtosha*), austerity (*tapas*), study (*svadhyaya*), and surrender to the Lord (*ishvara-pranidhana*)

Nazim: a courier of the court who serves notices.

Non-Being Essentiality: a word coined by the Yogiraj Siddhanath; this word is a paradox because *Para Brahma* is so beyond mortal conception that He is a Non-Being as far as we are concerned; and yet He is the essentiality of the very fabric of our Soul-essence and Creation.

O

ojas: 'vitality', the subtle energy produced through practice, especially the discipline of chastity (*brahmacharya*).

Omkar: the primordial sound and birthing hum of creation heard by the yogi in meditation and harnessed to evolve himself to evermore refined spheres of consciousness; the symbol of the reality in creation.

Ot-prot Surya: 'solar osmosis', solar *pranayam* originated by Yogiraj Siddhanath whereby the light energy of the sun (*prana*) is inhaled into the Self & the self is exhaled into the sun.

P

pada: feet. In devotion it is the lotus feet (charan kamal) of the Sadguru

palkhi: 'palanquin', mode of transport involving chairs

Pancha Mahabhutic Sharir: the physical body composed of the five elements of earth, water, fire, air, and ether.

pani: water

Para-Mukta Avadhoot: a supremely liberated state.

Para-Prakriti: superior subtle nature

Paramatman: 'Supreme Self', the Universal Self, which is singular, as opposed to the individuated self (*jiva-atman*) the divine indweller that exists in countless numbers of living beings, name for God.

paramahansa: 'supreme swan', having crossed the 4th level of initiation of a yogi; an honorific title which was given to great adepts, such as Ramakrishna and Yogananda now evolved beyond that stage.

Paramartha Satya: Supreme Truth beyond understanding.

Paras Mani: 'mercury gem'; mercury consolidated by alchemical process.

parinam: 'transformation', denoting the serial transformation of mind-purification; and simultanious expansion of consciousness as it awares itself from grosser to subtler & vaster dimensions of mind, a term in Patanjali's *Yoga Sutras*

Patanjali: Divine master of yoga who authored the *Yoga-Sutras*.

Pinda Brahmanda: the philosophy 'as in the self so in the universe;' eg. the human womb reflecting the cosmic matrix (matrika-divine womb).

pingala-nadi: 'sun channel', the *prana* current ascending on the right side of the central channel (*sushuma-nadi*) and associated with the sympathetic nervous system and having an energizing effect on the mind when activated; *see also ida nadi* 'moon channel'

Prajna: 'wisdom', the opposite of spiritual ignorance (*ajnana, avidya*)

Prajna paramita: knowledge to cross the river of samsara (gnosis).

Prakriti: 'creatrix', nature, which is multilevel and, according to Patanjali's *Yoga-Darshana*, consists of an eternal dimension or foundation (*pradhana*), levels of subtle existence (called *sukshma-parvan*), and the physical realm (called *sthula-parvan*); **prakriti nature is deemed unconscious, and therefore viewed as being lifeless without the 'Purusha' the Supreme Spirit**

prana: the upward flowing life-force energy in the spine; also the universal life enrgy animating the whole of creation, the breath of the Cosmic *Parusha*; in *Kriya Yoga* it is used for the evolution of human consciousness.

Pranapat: a term coined by Yogiraj Siddhanath to denote the grace of a *Sat-Guru*, when he breathes through the breath of the disciple; see also *shaktipat, shivapat.*

Pranayama: 'life-breath extension', breath control and expansion, the fourth limb (*anga*) of Patanjali's eightfold path, consisting of conscious inhalation (*puraka*), retention (*kumbhaka*), and exhalation (*rechaka*); at an advanced state, breath retention occurs spontaneously and for prolonged periods of time.

Prasava: breathing forth also known as faulty breathing.

Pratyaksha Daivam: emphasis that self realization is not knowledge based on any sensory input but direct perception acquired through self effort.

Prasada: 'grace/clarity', divine grace, mental clarity; food consecrated by the Guru or a deity.

pratyahara: 'withdrawal', sensory inhibition, the fifth limb (*anga*) of Patanjali's eightfold path.

puja: 'worship', prescribed rituals usually accompanied by the recitation of *mantras* or *shlokas*, an important aspect of many forms of *Yoga*, notably *Karma* and *Bhakti Yoga*

pujari: The priest who performs the temple rituals and prayers.

punarjamma: rebirth

puraka: 'filling in', inhalation, an aspect of breath control (*pranayama*)

Purana: the ancient spiritual literature of India dealing with royal genealogy, cosmology, philosophy etc., akashik recordings for a day of Brahma, there are eighteen major and many minor works of this nature.

Purusha 'male', the transcendental Self (*atman*) or Spirit, a designation that is mostly used in *Samkhya* and *Patanjali's Yoga-Darshana*.

Purshartha: 'human purpose' the four efforts for which people are responsible to pursued. These are *arth* (material welfare), *kama* (procreation), *dharma* (moral way of life) and *moksha*, (liberation).

Prakriti: casual matter, shakti also known as nature or creation.

R

raga: passion or attachment.

Radha: the Avatar Krsna's spouse; a name of the Divine Mother

Rainbow Body: 'radiant body', the body of the *Nath Yogi* who has transmuted his body-cells into the spectrum aura of light; *see kaya kalpa*

Raja Yoga: 'Royal Yoga', a late medieval designation of *Patanjali's* eightfold *yoga-darshana,* also known as Classical Yoga

Rama: an *avatar* of Vishnu preceding Krsna; the principal hero of the *Ramayana.*

Ramayana: '*Rama's* life' one of India's two great national epics telling the story of *Rama*; cf. *Mahâbhârata.*

rechaka: 'expulsion' exhalation, an aspect of breath control (*pranayama*).

reincarnation: '*Punar Janma*', the individual Soul rotating in the repeatd cycle of birth, death (the *kala chakra*) owing to bondage creating *karma.*

Rig-Veda: the most ancient literature and knowledge passed down from pre-history; *see also Veda*

rishi: 'seer', the Vedic Sages of the ancient of days; eg. some of the Brahma Rishi are Marich, Atri, Angiras, Pulastya, Bhrigu, Vashishta and Vishvamitra, an honorific title for venerated masters and Cosmic Beings.

S

sadhana: 'accomplishing', spiritual discipline leading to 'perfection' or 'accomplishment' (*siddhi*).

sahaja: 'together-born', natural enlightenment; the fact that the transcendental reality and the empirical reality are not truly separate but coexist, or with the latter being an aspect or misperception of the former; often rendered as 'spontaneous' or 'spontaneity'; the *sahaja* state is the natural condition, that is, enlightenment or realization.

samadhi: 'putting together', the ecstatic or unitive state in which the meditator becomes one with the object of meditation; the eighth and final limb (*anga*) of Patanjali's eightfold path; there are many types of *samadhi*, the most significant distinction being between *samprajnata* (super-conscious) and *asamprajnata* (supra-conscious) ecstasy; only the latter leads to the dissolution of the *karmic* factors deep within the mind; beyond both types of ecstasy is enlightenment, which is also sometimes called *sahaja-samâdhi* or the condition of 'natural' or 'spontaneous' ecstasy, where there is perfect continuity of supra-conscious throughout waking, dreaming, and sleeping

samatva: 'evenness', the mental condition of harmony, balance.

samkhya: 'number', one of the main philosophies of Yoga, which is concerned with the classification of the principles (*tattva*) of existence and their proper discernment in order to distinguish between Spirit (*Purusha*) and the various aspects of nature (*prakriti*); grew out of the ancient *Samkhya Yoga* tradition and was codified in the *Samkhya-Karika* of Ishvara Krishna 3000BCE.

samnyasa: 'casting off', the state of renunciation, which is the fourth and final stage of life (see *ashram*) and consisting primarily in an inner turning away from what is understood to be finite and secondarily in an external letting go of finite things; see *vairâgya*

samnyasin: 'he who has cast off', a renunciate

samprajnata-samadhi: *samadhi* with seed savikalpa samadhi

samsara: 'confluence', maya also jagat the finite world of change, as opposed to the ultimate reality (*Brahman*).

samskara: 'activator', a stored impression left behind by each act of volition/thought, which, in turn, leads to renewed psychomental activity; the countless *samskaras* hidden in the depth of ones memory banks began tobe eliminated in *asanprajnata-samadhi* (temporary seedless *samadhi*)

samyama: 'constraint', the combined practice of concentration (*dharana*), meditation (*dhyana*), and ecstasy (*samadhi*) in regard to the same object.

Sanctum Sanctorium: 'holiest of holies', the inner sanctum representing the womb or divine matrix.

sanjeevani: the yogic process of bringing others back to life. Ressurecting their physical body, for specific spiritual work.

Sanskrit: an ancient language said to have been brought by the *Rishis* from Venus and Sirius.

Sapta Rishi: the Seven Primordial Sages, corresponding to the seven stars of the Great Bear.

sat: 'truth', the ultimate reality (*Atman* or *Brahman*)

satguru: 'one with gravity', a Master who brings to light the Spiritual knowledge inherent in man; an enlightened aspect of the Divine

satsang: 'fellowship of Truth', the practice of frequenting the good company of saints, sages, Self-realized adepts, and their disciples; mentioned in the *Yoga Vashisht* as one of the four cornerstones to spiritual success.

satya: 'truth', a designation of the ultimate reality; also the practice of truthfulness, which is an aspect of moral discipline (*yama*).

satyagraha: 'truth grasper', nonviolent resistance to injustice in reference to Mahatma Gandhi.

sevak: a servant of humanity; a *hamsasevak* is one who has received the 1st level of initiation at the Hamsa Yoga Sangh.

shakti: 'power', the kinetic aspect of the potential Shiva (God-realization), the power to transform and evolve aspirants to this enlightened state; *see also kundalini shakti.*

shaktipat: 'descent of *shakti*', one of the three blessings (*shivapat*, *shaktipat*, and *pranapat*) SatGurunath bestows upon his disciples for their spiritual progress; the awakening of the dormant *kundalini* energy of a disciple.

Shambalpur: *Shamballa* also *Shangrilla*, where an aspect of Shiva-Goraksha-Babaji reigns as Sanat Kumar the Spiritual King until the world cycle is over; its higher center is in the Aurora Borealis of the Northern Lights.

shishya: 'chela/disciple', the initiated disciple of a Guru.

Shiva: 'the Benevolent One', the Consciousness of the universe. The great destroycr of delusion and spiritual rejenerator of mankind. He is the divine potential aspect of his own kinetic *shakti* energy; also called *Mahadeva* 'Great God.'

shiva netra: the third-eye chakra; also the third eye of Shiva, the location of the Hamsa swan seen visually in meditation. Kutastha Chaitanya.

shivapat: '*Shiva's* grace', the *Sat-Guru*, as Consciousness, awares himself into the mind-disciple, transforming that mind into his own Consciousness to the degree of the disciple's receptivity to his Consciousness; see also

pranapat, shaktipat.
Shiva Sutra: 'Shiva's Aphorisms', like the *Yoga-Sutra* of Patanjali, a classical work on Yoga, as taught in the *Shaivism* of Kashmir; authored by Vasugupta (ninth centuryCE)
shloka: a verse of praise, generally consisting of 32 letters. *see also mantra.*
shodhana: 'cleansing/purification', a fundamental aspect of all yogic paths; a category of purification practices in *Hatha Yoga.*
shraddha: 'faith', an essential disposition on the yogic path, which must be distinguished from mere belief.
shuddhi: 'purification/purity', the state of purity; see also *shodhana.*
Shveta Varaha Kalpa: 'World-Cycle of the White Boar.'
Shvetdeep: 'White Island' *see Shambalpur.* Residence of the spiritual King Sanat Kumar an aspect of Shiva-Gorakshya-Babaji. An astrocausal realm.
siddha: 'accomplished', a perfected Master or adept; a 5th degree initiate *mahasiddha* or 'great adept' from 6th to 7th degree initiates.
Siddha Sangh: a collective body of yogis who have taken the 5th degree of initiation; they are said to reside at a location in the Himalayas called Kalapa Gram; they form the *Guardian Wall of Humanity* to protect us from negative forces hitting our planet, protecting our nervous system, astral chakras, and boosting our evolution.
siddhi: 'accomplishment/perfection', spiritual perfection, the attainment of flawless identity with the ultimate reality (*atman* or *brahman*); paranormal ability, of which the Yoga tradition knows many kinds.
Sphurti Vada: doctrine of spontaneous manifestation
stitha-pradnya: 'he who is steadied in wisdom', the sage who is content abiding in the Self alone, who has expelled all desire and is neither dismayed by sorrowful events nor elated by joyous experiences.
sthula sharir: our gross physical bodies.
sukha: joy, pleasure or ease
Surya Narayana: the higher informing spirit of our visible sun.
Suryavanshi: descended from the sun. Tracing ones lineage to the sun.
sushumna-nadi: 'very gracious channel', the central *prana* current in or along which the serpent power (*kundalini shakti*) must ascend toward the psycho-energetic center (*chakra*) at the crown of the head in order to attain liberation (*moksha*).
sutra: 'thread', an aphoristic statement; a work consisting of aphoristic statements, such as Patanjali's *Yoga-Sutras* or Vasugupta's *Shiva-Sutra*
svadhyaya: self-study of purifying mind and expanding consciousness, in the yogic path, and Kriya Yoga in Patanjali's eightfold Yoga; the recitation of *mantras* and *japa* also a process of mind purification.

swami: 'owner' or 'lord', title of respect for a spiritual personage.

swaroop: (*svaroop*) embodiment of one's true Self; the essential nature of a thing

Swashan-Jwala: 'Breath of Fire', a *pranayama* technique of *Hamsa Yoga* involving the forceful breathing through each nostril and the mouth.

swayambhoo: 'great unborn', the self-manifestation and personal aspect of Lord Shiva. The cosmic being Babaji-Gorakshanath will not incarnate from age to age, but is perpetually present until the world cycle (*mahakalpa*) is over. His work is far beyond the comprehension of mortals; *Anupadaka* meaning self born in the world without human intervention.

T

tanmatra: 'fine astral matter', corresponding to the material elements (*bhutas*) which may be seen in the form of light during *yoni-mudra*; the potentials of sound (*shabda*), form (*rupa*), touch (*sparsha*), taste (*rasa*), and smell (*gandha*).

tantra: 'warp', the tradition of Tantrism and practice of tantric rights by which the laws of nature are manipulated and overcome; the esoteric and arcane practices of *sadhus* in India by which the *sadhak* may attain spiritual powers (*siddhis*) by means of *tantric* practice and *tapa*.

Tantra Aloka: Abhinav Gupta's magnum opus, which discusses in great depth the metaphysics and spiritual practice of Tantrism from the viewpoint of Kashmir Shaivism. Disciple of Matsendranath.

Tapah: 'glow' or 'heat', self directed austerity, an element of all yogic approaches, to loosen the grip which the body and the mind have on the soul; in yogic meditation, the act of stewing in one's own *pranic* energies thereby transforming one's body into the radiant body.

Tapasvi: '*Tapasvin*', a practicioner of *tapah*, the endurance of extremes, self directed austerity.

Tattva: 'thatness', a fact or reality; a particular category of existence such as the *ahamkara*, *buddhi*, *manas*; the ultimate reality; *see also atman*, *Brahman*.

teeka: a sacred mark worn by devotees at their third-eye center, made of processed tumeric, sandal wood paste or bhasma (holy ash).

Turiya: 'fourth', also called *Cathurtha* 'the transcendental reality' which exceeds the three conventional states of consciousness, namely waking, sleeping, and dreaming.

U

Unmani: a clear-mind ecstasy of thoughtless awareness.

Upanishad: 'sitting near', a classical Indian scripture representing the conclusion of the 'revealed literature' of *Sanatana Dharma* (the *Vedas*), hence the designation *Vedanta* for the teachings of these sacred works; *see also Aranyaka, Brahmana, Veda*

V

Vaidhatra: 'lightening holder', unborn manifestation of the Creator; Master of destiny; holder of the *Cosmic Kundalini*; a name of Shiva-Goraksha Babaji.

Vairagya: 'dispassion', the attitude of inner renunciation, the counterpole to *abhyasa*.

Vak: 'the word', divine sound with the resonant power of manifestation. Matrika mother gives birth to four sounds; *vaikhari* (loud sound), *madhyama* (murmuring sound), *pashyanti* (mental sound), *para* (meditative unheard sound); a name of **Sarasvati- Vak (sound) cf Brahma-Viraj (light)***cf Shabda cf Shabad* (a mis pronunciation) but all the same

Varuna: the deity presiding over the element of water and the oceans.

Vasana: 'trait', the constellation of subliminal activators (*samskara*) deposited in the depth of the mind where they exert a binding effect.

Vastu Gyan: the science of geomancy involving the proper directions for architecture: homes, temples, buildings, *etc*; attributed to *Vishvakarma*, the architect of the Gods. The Chinese took these ancient Indian records and translated them into the science *Feng-Shui*.

Vastuspati Shiva: the planet Sirius; the hunter (*Vyad*) who slays the deer (*Mrugnakshatra*, the constellation Orion). From this originated the science of *Vastu Gyan* "geomancy."

Vasudeva: 'Deva residing in the hearts of all beings'. Epiteth of Krsna

Vayu: the Hindu deity presiding over the element of wind.

Veda: 'knowledge', the body of sacred wisdom found in the four Vedic hymnodes that form the source of Hinduism: *Rig-Veda, Yajur-Veda, Sama-Veda,* and *Atharva-Veda*; also the collective name for these hymnodies; *see also Vedanta*

Vedanta: 'Veda's end', the teachings forming the doctrinal conclusion of the revealed literature (*shruti*) of *Sanatana Dharma*; *see also Upanishad*; cf. *Aranyaka, Brahmana, Veda*

videha-mukti: 'disembodied liberation', the state of liberation without a physical or subtle body; *see also jivan-mukti*

vidya: 'knowledge' or 'wisdom', a synonym of *prajna.*

Vigyan Bhairava: the supreme state of Consciousness, which is none other than Shiva.

Viraj-Vach: are Brahma-Sarasvati transformed to 'light-sound' respectively

Vishnu: 'pervader', the preserver; worshipped by *Vaishnavas* and who has had nine incarnations, including Rama and Krsna, with the tenth incarnation (*avatara*) Kalki coming at the start of the Leo-Aquarian age.

viveka: 'discernment', the aspect of the yogic path involving discrimination between the Self and the not-self (truth and falsehood)

vritti: 'whirl', in Patanjali's *Yoga-Darshana*, specifically the five types of mental activity: valid cognition (*pramana*), misconception (*viparyaya*), imagination (*vikalpa*), sleep (*nidra*), and memory (*smriti*)

vyakta: the properties of an object pertaining to the present

Vyasa: 'arranger', the name of several great sages, but specifically referring to Veda Vyasa, who arranged the Vedic hymns in their current form and who also is attributed with the compilation of the *Puranas,* the *Mahabharata*, and other works, including the commentary on the *Yoga-Sutras* of Patanjali, the *Yoga-Bhashya.*

Y

yajna: 'sacrifice', ritual fire sacrifice involving the chanting of *mantras* and *shlokas*. Yoga also knows of an inner sacrifice of kindling the internal flame of *kundalini.*

Yajnavalkya: the most renowned sage of the early *Upanishadic* era.

yama: 'discipline', the first limb (*anga*) of Patanjali's eightfold path, comprising moral precepts that have universal validity (such as non-harming and truthfulness); the name of the gatekeeper of the netherworld, Yama 'The First Mortal.'

yantra: 'device', a geometric design representing the body of one's meditation deity, used for external and internal concentration and worship

Yoga: 'union', the spiritual tradition and practice of uniting the individual soul (*Jiva*) with the Supreme Spirit (*Shiva*) origiinating in India; the unitive discipline by which inner freedom is sought; spiritual practice, as practiced in Hinduism, Buddhism, and Jainism, and transcending the entrapment of religious identification.

Yoga Anushasan: the Yoga of self administration.

Yoga Darshana: 'Yoga sight', Patanjali's *Raja-Yoga*

Yoga Sutra: 'Aphorisms of Yoga', Patanjali's aphoristic compilation forming a source of *Raja-Yoga*

Yogachara School: the Tarak Raj Yoga system expounded by Aaryasangh, a follower of Kalki-Maitreya, blessed by Shiva-Goraksha Babaji.

yogacharya: an adept of Yoga capable of teaching others.

Yogarudh: one astride the Yoga science, an adept in Yogasamadhi.

yogi: a male practitioner of Yoga

yogini: a female practitioner of Yoga

Yogiraj: 'King of Yogis', a title of exaltation and praise granted to a spiritual Master.

yoni: the female genitalia; also a symbol for the the supreme Goddess and source of the universe, the primordial deep; *see also linga*

yoni mudra: also known as *jyoti mudra* and *shan-mukhi-mudra*, the blocking of one's ears, eyes, and nostrils with one's fingers where the inner sound, *anahata-nada* (*omkar*) is heard and the soul star of light is seen at the third eye. Penetrate the stargate to enter *Nirvikalpa Samadhi*.

yuga: 'age', a division of time; as expounded by Swami Sri Yukteswar, the four ages of ascending and descending arcs (12,000 years in length), forming one *Mahayuga* of 24,000 years.

Index

A

H

L

N

O

P

S

Also available:

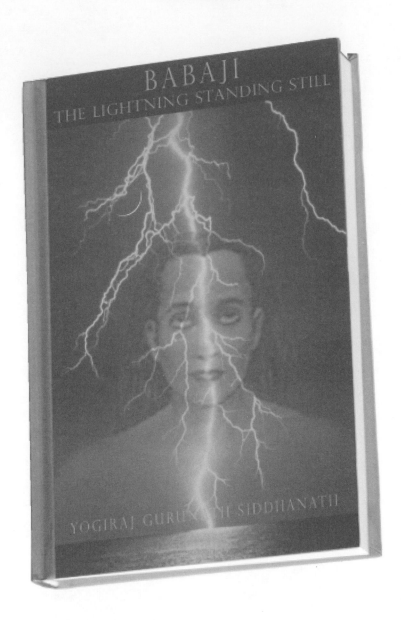

http://www.hamsayogashop.com

For more information on Yogiraj and Hamsa Yoga Sangh visit:

http://www.hamsa-yoga.org

http://www.youtube.com/hamsayogi